CARE OF PATIENTS WITH EMOTIONAL PROBLEMS

CARE OF PATIENTS WITH
EMOTIONAL PROBLEMS

DOLORES F. SAXTON, R.N., B.S., M.A., Ed.D.

Chairman and Professor of Nursing, Nassau Community College,
Garden City, N.Y.

PHYLLIS W. HARING, R.N., B.S., M.S., Ed.D.

Professor of Nursing, Nassau Community College,
Garden City, N.Y.

THIRD EDITION

The C. V. Mosby Company

ST. LOUIS · TORONTO · LONDON   1979

THIRD EDITION

Copyright © 1979 by The C. V. Mosby Company

All rights reserved. No part of this book may be reproduced in any manner without written permission of the publisher.

Previous editions copyrighted 1971, 1975

Printed in the United States of America

The C. V. Mosby Company
11830 Westline Industrial Drive, St. Louis, Missouri 63141

Library of Congress Cataloging in Publication Data

Saxton, Dolores F
    Care of patients with emotional problems.

    Bibliography: p.
    Includes index.
    1. Psychiatric nursing. I. Haring, Phyllis W.,
joint author. II. Title. [DNLM: 1. Nursing,
Practical. 2. Psychiatric nursing. WY160.3 S273c]
RC440.S33 1979   610.73′68   78-31641
ISBN 0-8016-4341-4

VT/M/M 9 8 7 6 5 4 3 2 1   03/B/343

Preface

This text has been planned to assist students of basic nursing in identifying and meeting the emotional needs of patients. The material in Part one provides students with background knowledge of the role that emotions play, so they can better understand their own behavior as well as the behavior of their patients. In Parts two and three, we have presented those situations most commonly encountered in the general hospital. By pointing out the obvious, we hope to encourage students to look for the less obvious and apply this knowlege in planning patient care. Although Part four is devoted to psychiatry, the concepts of psychiatric nursing are applicable to all interpersonal situations. We believe that a clearer understanding of the dynamics of behavior will remove some of the fears associated with the care of emotionally disturbed patients, and we sincerely hope this book will accomplish that goal.

In this third edition, among other changes we have expanded the material on personality development, crisis intervention, community psychiatry, and medications for mental illness. We have also added a chapter on remotivation through the use of groups. We hope the study questions at the end of each chapter will assist the student in reviewing and applying the material that has been presented.

Dolores F. Saxton
Phyllis W. Haring

Contents

Introduction, 1

Part one

THE EMOTIONAL DEVELOPMENT OF MAN

1 The parts of the personality, 11

2 Essential periods in the formation of the personality, 14

3 The role of anxiety, 25

4 The use of defense mechanisms, 30

5 Communication, 34

Part two

THE RELATIONSHIP BETWEEN PHYSICAL ILLNESS AND EMOTIONAL PROBLEMS

6 Patients with emotional problems resulting from physical illness, 41

7 Patients with physical illness resulting from emotional problems, 52

Part three

PATIENTS WITH EMOTIONAL DISORDERS

8 Patients with psychoneurotic disorders, 59

9 Patients with personality disorders, 66

10 Patients with addictive disorders, 70

Contents

Part four

PATIENTS WITH FUNCTIONAL PSYCHOTIC ILLNESSES

11 Tools utilized in psychiatric nursing, 79
12 Patients with schizophrenic reactions, 89
13 Patients with affective reactions, 102
14 Remotivating the emotionally disturbed patient through groups, 109

Bibliography, 113

Glossary, 118

Introduction

, During the past four decades the fields of psychiatry and nursing have both undergone vast changes. During World War II and the postwar period psychiatry advanced from its primitive stage of patient abuse, confinement, and isolation to the present-day interpersonal approach; during the same period the concept of nursing changed from that of the handmaiden to that of the skilled team member.

The behavioral differences of people suffering from what is now identified as psychiatric disorders were recognized in the earliest civilizations, but the reasons for such behavior were beyond comprehension and many superstitions were developed as explanations. The patients were frequently considered to be possessed by demons who had invaded their bodies to punish them for wrongdoings. The treatment consisted of rather severe and brutal methods. Needless to say, the cure was often worse than the disease, and many patients failed to survive the treatment. Those who did survive were frequently shocked back to reality and were therefore considered to be freed of the demon.

The Greek civilization ushered in some changes in the care of the mentally ill patient. The Greeks believed that Hera, wife of Zeus and Queen of Heaven, had the power to cause mental illness. Individuals with mental disorders were considered rather holy and were taken to temples, which were used as hospitals, for remedial treatment, which consisted of kindness, occupation, music, and recreation. Massage, friction, hydrotherapy, and hypnotism were also utilized in the treatment program. Hippocrates, the Greek physician, believed that all diseases had bodily causes and that mental illnesses resulted from excessive bile in the body. Plato, the Greek philosopher, believed that mentally ill people should not be allowed to walk in the city, but he believed that the relatives of these people had the responsibility of watching over them and caring for them in the best manner possible.

During the early Christian period there was a return to the superstitions of witchcraft and possession by demons as explanations for mental illness. The only difference between their attitudes and primitive attitudes was that the Christians considered it a sacred duty to care for the sick; therefore those who were strong and healthy cared for those who were weak and sick. Three methods were employed by the Christians to drive the demons from a patient's body: (1) a priest touched the patient and repeated a holy formula in the hope that the holy words and touch would be so disagreeable that the demons would leave; (2) the demons were addressed, shouted at, and talked to in a disrespectful manner in the hope that their pride would be offended and they would leave; and (3) the demons were tortured and punished in the hope that they would leave. This last method once again resulted in the abuse and actual death of many patients who were unable to survive the treatment.

The later Christian era, guided by St. Augustine, saw a return to a more humane treatment program. The sick were cared for in the monasteries, where kindness in patient care was assured. During this period dungeons were cleaned, beatings were forbidden, environmental stimuli were reduced, and diversional activities were recommended for the mentally ill person. When religious orders gave over the control of the mentally ill patients to lay groups, care once again degenerated into abuse. Belief in witchcraft prevailed, and seizures or deviant behaviors were considered positive proof of possession by demons.

Strange practices were used in attempts to cure patients and free them from their demons. For example, certain wells were considered to have curative powers; people who were thought to have demons infesting their heads were dunked, head first, three times into one of these wells. If they were not dunked, their heads were held under the water for a time. After the treatment they were bound and left till the next morning. If they freed themselves during the night, they were considered cured. If they died or were unable to free themselves, they were considered hopeless cases possessed by very powerful and unbeatable demons. Another method used to rid the body of demons consisted of lowering the patient into a pit of snakes; this was an attempt to scare the demons out of the "possessed" individual. In reality it frequently succeeded in scaring the patient to death and is considered the origin of the term *snake pit* frequently associated with poor psychiatric hospitals.

In 1247 the first large hospital for the care of mentally ill patients, Bethlehem Asylum, was opened in London. The word *asylum* meant "a place safe from violence," but later was used to specify institutions for the care of persons of unsound minds. The conditions at Bethlehem were so bad that the name, generally contracted to *Bedlam,* came to be a term that still means tumult or frenzy. The treatment of patients at Bethlehem was disgraceful; they were clothed in rags, slept on straw spread on the floor, and had deplorable sanitary facilities. They were chained to the walls of cells by iron collars and chains and were exhibited to the public who paid a small fee to watch the "entertaining" behavior. Those patients who were not considered violent were forced to beg in the streets for money to pay for their food and lodging.

The early pioneers in this country brought with them the fears and superstitions about mental illnesses that they had learned in their native countries, and the treatment of mentally ill patients was therefore the same. The Hotel Dieu, the first hospital on the American continent to care for mentally ill patients, opened in Quebec in 1639; none followed its lead for many years. Mentally ill patients were most often put into jails and treated as prisoners. In 1709 the Society of Friends of Philadelphia attempted to open a hospital that would accept mentally ill patients; but, even with the help and support of Benjamin Franklin, the Pennsylvania Hospital did not admit its first patient until 1752. Dr. Benjamin Rush, called the Father of American Psychiatry, later became director of this institution. His emphasis on humane treatment of patients and his beginning theories on the importance of occupational therapy did a great deal toward improving the lot of these patients.

3

In 1771 the New York Hospital was established, and a section for the treatment of "maniacs" was built in the basement. The area was very small and congested, had little sunlight or fresh air, and soon was totally overcrowded. In 1773 the first hospital exclusively for the care of mentally ill patients was opened in Williamsburg, Virginia. It is still in operation and is now known as the Eastern State Hospital.

Poor conditions existed in most hospitals for mentally ill patients until the work of Philippe Pinel in France, William Tuke in England, and Benjamin Rush and Dorothea Lynde Dix in America became known and accepted.

Pinel was a French physician who was named chief of the Bicetre Institution for Psychiatric Patients in France. At this "asylum" patients were kept in chains and were mistreated. Pinel felt that a great deal of their violence was the result of their being deprived of "light, liberty, and air." His action of removing the chains assured him a place of honor in the history of psychiatry. The first patient to be freed of his chains was an English captain. Having been chained for 40 years, he was considered the most dangerous patient in the institution. Pinel not only removed his chains, but permitted him to go out in the fresh air and sunlight. Much to everyone's surprise, the captain did no harm and returned to his cell of his own accord. Pinel had proved his point; as word of his work spread, treatment of these patients began to improve. Shortly after Pinel's results became known, William Tuke, a member of the Society of Friends, began a reform movement in England. He established the York Retreat at York; this institution became world renowned for its humane treatment of patients with mental illnesses. Tuke spent many years in attempting to rid mental institutions of the restraint method of treatment.

About this time Charles Dickens, the English author, began writing his many books on social injustice in England and the United States; Dorothea Lynde Dix, an American schoolteacher, became very interested in his work. While visiting a house of correction in Massachusetts, she found a number of mentally ill patients among the inmates. On further investigation of the Massachusetts penal system, she found this condition to be true in most of the penal institutions. Miss Dix spent the next 20 years conducting this type of investigation throughout the country; in 1843 she presented a report to the United States Congress. As a result of her pressures, legislative action was secured and appropriations were provided for the building of several large state hospitals for mentally ill patients, many of which still exist. Her activities earned her the title of "patron saint of the insane" and assured her a place in any history of psychiatric care. It should be noted that none of Miss Dix's studies mentioned nursing care because at the time of her investigation nursing care for mentally ill patients was nonexistent.

During this same period psychiatrists such as Jean Martin Charcot of France, Emil Kraepelin of Munich, Eugene Bleuler of Zurich, Sigmund Freud of Vienna, and Adolph Meyer of Switzerland and later of the United States were all contributing to the development of the theory basic to the study of modern psychiatry. Although they produced material necessary to the understanding of mental illness, their work had very little effect on the care of the hospitalized psychiatric patient.

Dickens' works stimulated Miss Dix into action, and a book by Clifford Beers published in 1907, *A Mind that Found Itself,* stimulated society. Mr. Beers had been mentally ill and was confined in a psychiatric hospital prior to writing this book of his experiences. He came from a wealthy, influential family in Connecticut and used his influence and wealth to organize the Connecticut State Society for Mental Hygiene. This organization met with such success that, a year later, the National Society for Mental Hygiene was organized. Both of these organizations accomplished a great deal toward the opening of more hospitals and clinics for the care of mentally ill patients.

The public became aware of the need to support a state hospital system; the hospitals were constructed on large acreage away from the cities, where the patients could be locked up and yet have the fresh air and sunshine thought necessary for their well-being. Few patients were discharged from the system once they were admitted, but society felt it was providing a haven for its less fortunate members—as long as they were removed from view they could be forgotten. Perhaps the situation would have continued along in the same pattern for many more years had not certain factors intervened during the 1940s and 1950s.

One of the main factors was the massive call-up to meet the manpower needs of the military during World War II. Not only did state hospital care deteriorate as many of the better attendants were called into service, but the statistics that more than two million young men were rejected for service and another half million discharged from service because of neuropsychiatric problems really shocked and awoke the public to the immensity of the problem.

Another major factor was that the mass number of psychiatric casualties resulting from the war required the development of new and better methods of treatment. These young men could not be put out in the countryside and forgotten. Greater public understanding and acceptance of emotional problems resulted in a real desire to get involved and to reform and refine the old methods of treatment. As a result of this

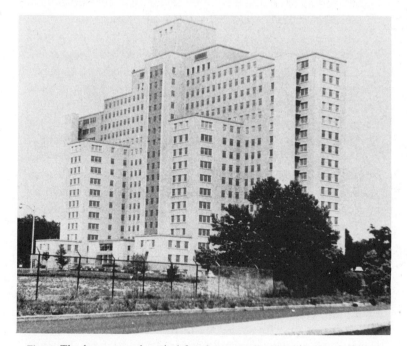

Fig. 1. The large state hospital for the mentally ill still appears on the horizon.

emphasis on treatment and research, the tranquilizing drugs were discovered, and the gates of many institutions opened to discharge patients who had been inside their doors for many years.

Still another factor was the mass exodus from the cities to the suburbs. The state hospitals, once far out in the country, were now in the backyards of the public, and the public began to accept them as neighbors.

The developments in the area of interpersonal relationships began to shift the emphasis from psychiatric patients to the emotional needs of all patients and their families. This shift required a change in focus from deviations in behavior to the prevention of emotional problems and the maintenance and promotion of mental health. The realization that psychiatric patients were simply patients with emotional problems and as such could be cared for by the general hospitals in the community, or even in the home, has completed the historical circle—from the earliest treatment at home, to the jails, to the general hospitals, to the asylums, back to the general hospital, and finally back to the home.

World War II can also be viewed as a milestone in the development of the nursing profession. The numbers of professional nurses required in the armed forces during the war created a severe shortage of nurses in many civilian hospitals. To meet their patients' needs, these hospitals began Cadet Nurse Programs, which increased the numbers of nurses entering the profession. The number of nurses graduating yearly has remained high since that time.

The role of the nurse in today's complex and confused medical care picture is sometimes hard to define. Although guidelines for education and practice are set by individual state-controlled nurse practice acts, nurses are frequently forced into situations that are unexpected and overwhelming. The student nurses' experiences on units of psychiatric institutions provide little incentive for working with emotionally disturbed patients after graduation. However, in today's community hospitals the graduate is often faced with caring for emotionally disturbed patients on general medical-surgical units. The attitudes acquired as a student greatly influence

7

functioning as a graduate. If these attitudes are not altered by education and experience, emotionally ill patients stand little chance of receiving the necessary acceptance and nursing care.

It is an accepted fact that the soma cannot be separated from the psyche; the body and mind act as a whole. If studies have repeatedly demonstrated that satisfied emotional needs make a difference in the recovery rate of psychiatric patients, it can be assumed that satisfied emotional needs can make a difference in the recovery rate of all patients. Making this objective a reality is the major objective of this book.

Part one

THE EMOTIONAL DEVELOPMENT
OF MAN

CHAPTER 1

The parts of the personality

Conscious, subconscious, and unconscious

Emotional development begins with the first breath of life and continues until the last. People are social beings who are continually reacting with and attempting to control their emotional environment. Behavior is a learned response, developed as a result of all past experience; in an attempt to protect the emotional well-being, the psyche organizes thoughts about these past experiences into three distinct levels—the conscious, the subconscious, and the unconscious.

The conscious level of thought is composed of those past experiences and related emotions that are easily recalled to mind and create little if any emotional discomfort when brought to complete awareness. Although a great deal of material remains at the conscious level, it is only a small part of the human psyche.

The subconscious level of thought is composed of those past experiences and related emotions that have been rather deliberately pushed out of the conscious level but that can be recalled to awareness. The emotions related to these experiences have usually created some emotional discomfort, and frequently this discomfort will again be felt when the material is brought back into the conscious level. The recall of subconscious material can be the result of a deliberate desire to remember an incident, or can occur spontaneously when a current experience brings to mind a similar situation from the past.

The unconscious level of thought contains the largest body of material and is composed of those past experiences and related emotions that have been completely removed from the

11

conscious level. Although the material in the unconscious greatly influences the individual's behavior, it cannot be readily brought back to a level of awareness. The past experiences and feelings relegated to the unconscious level are usually unacceptable to the conscious self and have been associated with situations that created severe emotional disturbance and discomfort for the individual. In an attempt to at least partially protect the individual from this emotional discomfort, any material leaving the unconscious is brought back to awareness in a disguised and distorted form. However, even though the actual experience is recalled in a disguised and distorted form, the feelings and emotions associated with the original experience cannot be disguised or distorted and usually create the same degree of emotional discomfort as they did in the past.

Man is the only animal capable of this process of sorting and organizing thoughts and the psyche. Although these processes contribute to and appear necessary for man's emotional survival, they do seem to predispose to certain emotional illnesses that cannot be found or produced in any other animal.

Id, ego, and superego

According to Freud, the personality consists of three parts—the id, the ego, and the superego. These names are used to designate the different functions within the personality. This breakdown of the personality is an imaginary division and cannot be measured or observed except by the individual's behavioral responses. The balanced operation of the id, the ego, and the superego contributes to the overall picture of the well-adjusted person.

The id is that part of the personality that contains the instincts, impulses, and urges and operates almost totally at the unconscious level of thought. It is believed that the id is the first part of the personality to be formed and that it supplies the newborn with the drive for survival. Some examples of id drives include hunger, aggression, sex, protection, and warmth. The id operates on the pleasure principle and therefore demands almost immediate satisfaction of its drives.

The ego is that part of the personality that deals with the individual's relationships with the world. It is the personal reaction to the environment, the conscious self, the "I." It is through this part of the personality that sensations, thoughts, feelings, compromises, solutions, and defenses are formed. The ego begins to develop during the first 6 to 8 months of life and is usually fairly well developed by 2 years of age. The ego is concerned with the environment, for the purpose of achieving maximum gratification for the id, within the scope of the pressures exerted by the superego.

The superego is that part of the personality that controls, inhibits, and regulates those impulses and instincts whose uncontrolled expression would endanger the stability of society. It is the collector of the parents' and society's moral and social codes. The superego starts developing by 3 or 4 years of age and is fairly well developed by 10 or 11 years of age. It is at this age that the values of the parents and society are internalized and become part of the individual's approach to life. The superego operates at both the conscious and unconscious levels of thought and helps the individual to decide what is right and what is wrong. The superego aids in critical self-evaluation, self-punishment, self-praise, and self-love.

It can be seen from these descriptions of the parts of the personality that the id is chiefly concerned with the individual's survival, the superego is chieflly concerned with society's survival, and the ego acts as a balance between instinctual drives and societal demands to produce an individual who can survive and function within the environment.

If these parts of the personality could speak, the conversation would probably follow these lines:

id—I want what I want when I want it.

superego—You can't have it.

ego—Why not wait to see what tomorrow brings.

Study questions

1. Dreams are frequently an expression of what level of thought?
2. Explain why simple incidents that occur in adulthood may trigger an exaggerated emotional response.
3. Explain why an individual's behavior may differ under tension.
4. What type of behavior would you expect to observe in an individual with an exceedingly strong superego?
5. What part of the personality is most often observed in others?

CHAPTER 2

Essential periods in the formation of the personality

The personality of the individual develops in overlapping stages. Certain goals must be accomplished during each stage in the development from infancy to maturity. If these goals are not accomplished, the structure of the personality will be weak; even if the psychologic growth is not completed, the chronologic growth will propel the individual into the next stage of development. Perhaps this concept can best be understood by comparing it with the construction of a brick wall. If one of the lower layers of brick is poorly constructed, the entire wall will have difficulty in standing if pressure is applied.

The psychologic development of the child follows the periods of physical development. For a clearer understanding, the following classification by ages will be used for these periods.

infancy—birth until 1 or 1½ years

toddler—1½ to 3 or 4 years

preschool—3 or 4 to 6 years

early school—6 to 9 years

preteen—9 to 12 years

early teen—12 to 16 years

late teen—16 to 20 years

adulthood—over 20 years

Infancy

The family, classified as the primary social group, serves as the milieu in which the socialization process begins. Those adults surrounding the child become significant figures in the development of the self-concept. The newborn's biologic equipment enables the infant to evaluate the emotional environment in a very limited manner, namely, through the satisfaction of oral needs and through physical contact. If the id drives, such as hunger, warmth, and comfort are met, the newborn feels accepted and wanted. The infant begins to have confidence in others; this basic confidence is the primary goal for this period.

Toddler

The child's self-concept continues to develop from the reflections seen in the eyes of others, and this self-concept controls both the willingness and ability to relate to others. The world of reality, that world of the parents, must demonstrate both pleasures and rewards if the child is expected to enter it, endure its failures and hurts, and abandon the gratifications of the self-centered inner world. This conflict is heightened during the toddler phase by the struggle with the parent over toilet training.

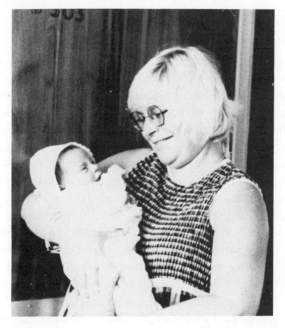

Fig. 2. Mother-child relationship—cornerstone for emotional security.

15

At this stage of development, children believe that to be loved is to be worthy of being loved. Since children are still totally dependent on the parental figures for their physical needs, they are forced to maintain an image of them as loving figures. In children's minds the concept exists that if they do not receive love it is not because the parents are not giving it, but rather because they are not worthy of receiving it. Only through developing this feeling of worth can they give of themselves to others. Children who feel rejected believe that they have nothing to offer others and tend to remain shut in rather than reaching out.

This period of development may be marked by conflict resulting from the toddler's early communication. As the toddler begins to move out independently, learning the word *no* long before the word *yes,* many problems with the parents occur, especially if the child's attempts at independence are met with rejection. The toddler's independent reaching out, although difficult at times, must be supported, for this independence is the primary goal of this period.

Preschool

The activities of the preschool period are designed to assist the child in exploring reality. Most of the preschooler's time is occupied by fantasy, imitation, and experimentation. In the male child's fantasy, he replaces his father in his mother's affection and secretly harbors a death wish for his father. Since his father does not usually disappear, he remains an unbeatable opponent, an opponent who is both hated and loved, unwanted but needed. The same pattern of development occurs in the female child during this period, except that the father becomes the love object and the mother becomes the opponent.

The child's experimentation with reality includes the exploration of the body, including the genital area. Masturbation, though a normal and natural phenomenon during this period, frequently brings the child into conflict with the parents' moral code. The secret desires and thoughts about both the mother and the father, in addition to this masturbation, create feelings of shame and guilt in the child. The child feels that there is

16   something unacceptable about these thoughts and actions and

fears that the parents will find out about them and punishment will occur. In an attempt to alleviate some of the guilt, the child completely imitates the behavior of the parent of the same sex, in reality becoming a little adult. Thus the moral codes of the parents and society are internalized and the growth of the superego is furthered.

The chief goals for this age group can be identified as the beginning acceptance of the life roles and the internalization of the parents' and society's values.

Early school

The independent strivings of the preschool period are magnified as children move out of the home and into the school. A great deal of the social activity moves by necessity from the family circle into the peer group. The trauma of this initial separation from the family may be intensified if the social standards of the peer group are greatly different from those already learned. This is a period of work, and children's work consists of learning to compete with and adjusting to the needs and desires of their own age group. They have to learn how to win recognition, for their teachers and their schoolmates may not accept their previous behavior, which was successful in the family. In this competitive society in which they find themselves there are frequently winners and losers, and children are forced to deal with both situations. The chief goal of this period is the accomplishment of a feeling of comfort and security within the peer group.

Preteen

The preteen period is one of intensified group activity, with groups composed exclusively of members of the same sex. The close relationships that are formed with members of the same sex during this period enable preteens to deal successfully with members of their own sex in competitive situations in later life.

There is a beginning restlessness and irritability with the family, and except for the basic physical needs, the child tends to abandon the family for the companionship of chums. The formation of clubs with secret rites is common, with group accomplishments bringing more satisfaction than individual achievements. The chief goal for this period is the replacement of the ego-centered "I" by the group-centered "we."

Early teen

The early teen period begins with the onset of puberty and is characterized by the intense struggle to become an adult. It is the time of overidentification with heroes, cliques, and crowds. There are great feelings of insecurity and inadequacy in fulfilling the role of the adult, for teenagers fear they may not measure up to their own idealized standards. The relationships in this age group move from members of the same sex to members of the opposite sex, and a great deal of activity is devoted to finding a suitable sexual object. The chief goal of this period is the establishment of satisfactory relationships with the opposite sex.

Late teen

The late teen period is characterized by those tasks associated with sex, education, and occupation. The teenager moves from broad general relationships with the opposite sex to a more durable and binding relationship with a single member. They are faced with making decisions that will greatly influence their future both economically and socially. Their future field of employment is frequently decided by their choice of schooling. The many choices forced on the teenager produce both tension and anxiety and create the typical picture of mood swings so common in this age group. Relief from these feelings is sought by some in experimentation with sex, drugs, and alcohol, but it should be noted that the majority of teenagers learn to tolerate the anxiety and use it constructively. The goal for this period is the formation of interdependent rather than independent relationships.

Adulthood

All people do not achieve adulthood emotionally, even if they achieve it chronologically. The criterion for emotional adulthood is maturity. This maturity may be evaluated by the following factors.

18   intelligence—The individual can use the intellect in ac-

cordance with reality; there is freedom from delusions, phobias, and hallucinations.

reality oriented—The individual is practical and straight-forward and does not spend time daydreaming. Stimulation is derived from realistic situations.

long-term goals—The individual has the ability to set long-term goals and can accept disappointments and frustrations in reaching them. There is recognition that the purpose of life is more than a search for pleasure.

sense of morality—The individual develops ethical principles. These principles are developed out of a sense of love for others rather than out of a fear of punishment.

independence—The individual is no longer dependent on the parents but develops and provides for a new family unit. There is freedom to make decisions but consideration is given to the effect those decisions will have on others.

love—The individual has the capacity to love and the ability to accept love. Sexual maturity reaches and remains at the heterosexual stage.

fear—Although the mature person experiences fear, it is in relationship to something real, and there is an ability to identify and act on the source of danger.

aggression—The mature individual expresses aggressive and hostile feelings that are healthy and necessary for survival. Aggression is exerted in proportion to the attack and is directed toward a real enemy.

The mature person has the ability to live life in relative harmony with the enviornment. The individual's demonstration of good reasoning and sound judgment results in an adequate social adaptation.

Tasks and activities of growth periods

The following section briefly outlines the tasks and activities included in the personality theories of Freud, Erikson, and Sullivan as they relate to the periods of growth. A brief summary of the nursing activities directed toward assisting the individual to accomplish the tasks of each period is also included.

19

INFANCY—MAJOR STRESS IS SURVIVAL

Freud (Birth to 1 year)	Erikson (Birth to 1 year)	Sullivan (Birth to 1½ years)
Oral stage Id functioning Mouth—taking in or biting off Symbiosis	Trust—feeling of inner goodness resulting from quality of maternal care Mistrust versus lack of trust in the caring one	Learning to count on others Beginning anxiety Security—satisfaction Empathy "Good me—bad me"

NURSING ACTIONS
1. Teach infant care—assist parents to relax.
2. Support family.
3. Keep separation from significant others as short as possible.
4. Encourage parents to provide care to hospitalized infant by living-in or assign same staff member to provide a consistent figure.

TODDLER—MAJOR STRESS IS LEARNING SELF-CONTROL

Freud (1-2 years)	Erikson (1-2 years)	Sullivan (1½-6 years)
Anal stage Ambivalence (love-hate) Magical thoughts Temper tantrums	Development of autonomous will If deprived of opportunity to learn, child will develop deep sense of shame and doubt and learn to expect defeat	Childhood language Learning to delay satisfaction Learning to use power Learning to accept interference

NURSING ACTIONS
1. Deemphasize stress of toilet training.
2. Provide or teach parents to provide for learning by:
   a. giving child opportunity for exploring
   b. giving child realistic praise for accomplishments
   c. minimizing "don'ts" while emphasizing "do's"
   d. setting limits allowing for alternative actions

20

PRESCHOOL—MAJOR STRESS IS DEVELOPING ROLE IDENTITY

Freud (3-5 years)	Erikson (3-5 years)	Sullivan (1¹/₂-6 years)
Oedipal stage Superego development Conflict—wishes to possess parent of opposite sex and reject parent of same sex—fears punishment for these feelings Resolution of conflict— identifies with parent of same sex	Play age Imagination greatly expanded Curiosity and fan- tasies lead to guilt if initiative is stifled by others Beginning of moral values	Body image Need to be like significant others

NURSING ACTIONS
1. Assist parents to understand child learns through play.
2. Help improve relationships between family members if problems exist.
3. Help parents understand that masturbation and the occurrence of nightmares are common in this period.
4. Help parents understand that child should be given the opportunity to explore the roles of both sexes.
5. Assist parents to answer child's sexual questions frankly.
6. Prepare child emotionally if surgery must be performed as fear of mutilation is overwhelming during this period.

CHILDHOOD—MAJOR STRESS IS DEVELOPING SOCIAL ROLE

Freud (6-12 years)	Erikson (6-12 years)	Sullivan (6-9 years)
Latency period Social achievement Balance of freedom and control	School age Wants to make things with others Accepts instruction and needs recog- nition to enjoy work Will feel inferior if recognition is not given	Peer groups Competition Learning compro- mise and coop- eration

NURSING ACTIONS
1. Encourage child to work with groups of own age.
2. Give praise and encouragement for efforts and accomplishments.
3. Provide a stimulating environment.
4. Set controls and limits that child can understand and accept.

PREADOLESCENCE—MAJOR STRESS IS LEARNING TO LOVE SOMEONE OF SAME SEX

Freud	Erikson	Sullivan (9-13 years)
Continuation of previous period	Continuation of previous period	Learns to care for members of same sex Learns to use consensual validation Learns to rely on group validation Most important phase of development

NURSING ACTIONS
1. Observe relationships with age mates, prevent isolation but permit secrecy.
2. Provide guidance to both child and family in preparation for puberty.

EARLY ADOLESCENCE—MAJOR STRESS IS DEVELOPING SEXUAL AND SELF-IDENTITY

Freud (12-18 years)	Erikson (12-18 years)	Sullivan (12-14 years)
Genital stage Daydreaming Hero worship Heterosexual versus homosexual role	Adolescence Rapid body growth Sexual maturity Earlier developmental problems reappear Need to integrate basic biologic drives, native endowment, and social role or there will be identity diffusion	Early adolescence Lust Fantasy Cliques Anxiety Moodiness Learning independence

NURSING ACTIONS
1. Encourage independence.
2. Provide family counselling to assist parents in setting limits while providing some degree of freedom.
3. Encourage physical exercise and group activities to discourage premature sexual expression.

YOUNG ADULTHOOD—MAJOR STRESS IS INTIMACY

Freud	Erikson (18-25 years)	Sullivan (14-21 years)
Does not cover this period	Establish intimacy with self and others Love of opposite sex If unable to develop intimate relationships, will develop sense of isolation	Learning to be independent Learning to deal with intimacy Learning how to release tension

ADULTHOOD—MAJOR STRESS IS PROVIDING FOR SELF AND OTHER

Freud	Erikson (25-65 years)	Sullivan
Does not cover this period	Generativity Interest in establishing and guiding the next generation, otherwise will become self-absorbed and stagnated	Does not cover this period

23

SENESCENCE—MAJOR STRESS IS LOSS OF SELF-IMAGE AND COMPANIONS

Freud	Erikson (65 years plus)	Sullivan
Does not cover this period	If person has established intimacy with others and has adapted to triumphs and disappointments, there will be ego integrity and acceptance of what life is and was— otherwise there will be despair and disgust	Does not cover this period

NURSING ACTIONS FOR YOUNG ADULTHOOD, ADULTHOOD, AND SENESCENCE
1. Meet dependent needs.
2. Support during crisis periods.
3. Provide for independence.

Study questions

1. What is the role of significant others in the formation of the personality?
2. Explain why excessive eating, drinking, or smoking in adulthood is believed to be related to problems in the infant stage of development.
3. What problems may result when toilet training is started before the child is physiologically ready?
4. Explain why play is a learning tool for the preschooler.
5. Compare the goals of adulthood with the other periods of development and explain how each of these periods contributes to the achievement of the goals of adulthood.

CHAPTER 3

The role of anxiety

The motivating factor in an individual's emotional life is the phenomenon of anxiety. Anxiety controls behavior to the extent that a person will usually take the course of action that will reduce the feelings of apprehension, tension, and uneasiness that originate from within and threaten the ego. These feelings stem from an anticipation of danger that may or may not be related to the reality of the present situation.

Anxiety is first experienced in infancy as a response to an interference with the gratification of needs. It continues throughout the life cycle of the individual, acting as either an assistance or a hindrance in the attainment of goals. The anxiety engendered in the early developmental periods frequently recurs when a present situation stimulates recall of a past situation that has been stored in the unconscious. The ego attempts to protect the individual by disguising and distorting any material leaving the unconscious. However, the feelings and emotions attached to the original situation cannot be successfully disguised or distorted, and they usually create the same degree of anxiety as they did in the past. These past feelings tend to exaggerate and intensify the anxieties in the present situation. This concept can best be demonstrated by the following example.

As a youngster, the child fails to wake up during the night, and in the morning the bed is wet. The mother severely chastises the child and states, "Nobody will like you if you don't stop doing this." The feelings and emotions associated with this incident are fear of rejection, fear of failure, and fear of abandonment. The incident and the associated fears and anxiety are repressed in the unconscious in an attempt to reduce the tension resulting from the situation. In later years, while studying for a final exam, these earlier fears are recalled by the present situation. Since the facts are disguised and distorted, the original situation is not recalled. This test is no longer a test of knowledge, but a test of the person's worth. The teacher is no longer a mere teacher, but is endowed with unlimited powers over the very life of the individual. The usual anxiety associated with test-taking is intensified by these earlier fears, and the importance of the testing situation is magnified completely out of proportion.

Anxiety can be experienced in various degrees, from the mild stage of apprehension to the severe stage of panic. Anxiety can occur or be relieved at any stage or can progress to the next level.

Mild anxiety or apprehension increases the person's alertness for a more efficient performance. There is a conscious awareness of some internal discomfort that may be accompanied by physical symptoms such as increased perspiration, dryness of the mouth, butterflies in the stomach, and increased heart rate. The individual may take a positive action such as studying to reduce the anxiety or may attempt to escape from the anxiety-producing situation through daydreams, making excuses, or even physically leaving the situation.

If the positive action or the attempt at escape is unsuccessful, the anxiety will tend to increase in severity to a more disorganized level. At this level the individual will begin to focus on many minute details as an escape from looking at the total situation. Reality is distorted and there are many fears and inhibitions. A feeling of impending doom develops, and the anxiety tends to become free-floating rather than being associated with a specific situation. Positive action to reduce this degree of anxiety is extremely difficult, if not impossible, and attempts to escape are limited to behavioral actions rather than thought mechanisms. Although the individual is usually aware of this behavior, there is usually little awareness of the factors that are motivating it. Some of the behavioral mechanisms used for escape include physical complaints of imaginary ill-

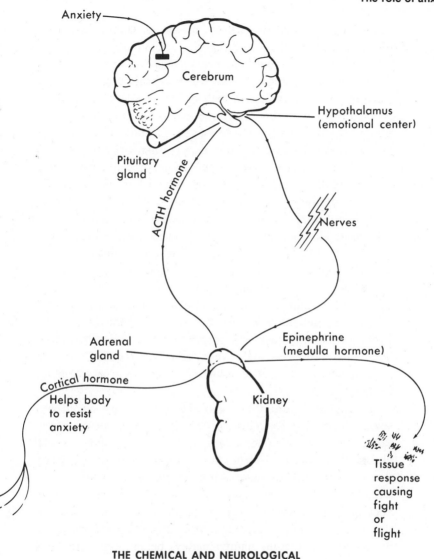

**THE CHEMICAL AND NEUROLOGICAL
PATH OF ANXIETY**

Fig. 3. Anxiety reaches the cerebrum and stimulates both the pituitary gland and the hypothalamus. This action results in 2 responses: (1) the pituitary gland excretes the ACTH hormone, which in turn stimulates the cortex of the adrenal gland, which then produces the cortical hormone to help the body resist anxiety; and (2) the hypothalamus sends out stimuli along the autonomic nervous system to the medulla of the adrenal gland, which then produces epinephrine and prepares the tissues for the fight or flight response.

27

ness, fears attached to persons, places, or things, obsessive thoughts, and ritualistic and repetitive actions.

If the behavioral mechanisms are unsuccessful in relieving the anxiety at this stage, the severely incapacitating, unrealistic stage of terror or panic will develop. At this level of anxiety, rational thought, action, and judgment are greatly impaired or totally absent. In an attempt to escape, the individual may race headlong into an even greater danger than originally faced. Many instances have been reported of persons jumping from a burning building just as the ladder was being placed at the window. Although the behavior during the stage of terror or panic is truly emotionally disturbed behavior, it can occur for a brief period in the emotionally stable individual. However, the emotionally stable person experiences the feelings as a response, even though it may be an exaggerated response, to reality. The emotionally disturbed person may experience this stage of terror and panic without relationship or accord to reality. Such an individual will frequently utilize behavior such as withdrawal into fantasy, inappropriate moods, disturbances in the thought processes, and severe regression to earlier levels of development as means of escaping from this overwhelming feeling of terror.

Perhaps a situation that many of us have experienced will serve to make this concept of progressive anxiety a bit clearer. You can recall getting home late one night and having to walk one block to your house from the bus stop. As you ride toward the stop, you think of that one-block walk and start developing a mild feeling of apprehension. You may begin to perspire and become aware that your heart is beating faster. As you leave the bus, your anxiety increases and you begin to pay a great deal of attention to the many shadows behind every tree and bush. Reality becomes distorted, and the once familiar neighborhood turns into a threatening maze. The nightmare may end here, or a slight swaying of the trees or the movement of a cat can send you into the stage of panic and result in your racing, unmindful of traffic or other real dangers, to your door.

Study questions

1. Recall a very anxious patient for whom you have cared. List the behaviors that helped you identify that the patient was anxious.

2. What different types of behavior may be observed in a group facing a common danger?
3. Trace the pathway of anxiety from the cerebrum to the tissue response.
4. Explain the role of anxiety in protecting an individual.
5. How does anxiety over past experiences affect our present emotional responses?

CHAPTER 4

The use of defense mechanisms

Defense mechanisms serve as an armor for the ego and are utilized by both the emotionally stable and the emotionally unstable individual; they serve to protect the personality by controlling anxiety and reducing emotional pressures. It is not the defense mechanism itself but the frequency of its use that may be unhealthy. Since the defense mechanisms are used to reduce anxiety, they play a major role in the behavioral responses of the individual. The nurse must recognize that these mechanisms are serving a useful purpose for the individual, and any attempt to interfere with their use will cause the individual to experience increased anxiety and tension.

Some of the more common mechanisms are the following.

compensation—The individual makes up for a felt lack in one area by emphasizing capabilities in another.

EXAMPLE: A young man who feels inferior in athletics develops exceptional skill in mathematics.

conversion reaction—An emotional conflict that is changed into a physical symptom without a physical cause is a conversion reaction. The person cannot get rid of the emotional conflict by the use of the thought processes, so it is changed into a physical symptom that can be expressed openly and without anxiety. It must be understood that this symptom is real to the person and is not classified as malingering.

EXAMPLE: A soldier in combat is scheduled to lead a night patrol and is anxious and fearful for his life. This fear

and the idea that he is acting like a coward are unacceptable thoughts to him and create an emotional
conflict. Unable to resolve the conflict, he develops a
very real symptom of blindness. He truly cannot see;
therefore he cannot lead the patrol.

denial—The individual refuses to recognize the reality of
an anxiety-producing situation.

EXAMPLE: A patient is told that the tests for cancer were
positive and surgery must be performed. The procedure
is thoroughly explained by the doctor. An hour later the
patient fails to remember that the doctor even visited.

displacement—A shifting of feelings from an emotionally
charged situation to a substitute person or object is
known as displacement. This usually occurs when the
expression of the emotions in the original situation
would be dangerous and threatening to the ego.

EXAMPLE: A doctor has just berated a nurse for not
carrying out an order. A visitor walks into a patient's
room. Without waiting to question the visitor, the nurse
abruptly and harshly tells him to leave and wait until
visiting hours.

fantasy—A conscious distortion of unconscious wishes or
needs is known as fantasy.

EXAMPLE: A young boy physically unable to defend his
mother from his father's attacks daydreams that his
home is besieged by a herd of wild animals and that
single-handed he kills them all, saving the family from
death.

identification—Identification is similar to imitation but occurs on an unconscious level. The individual internal-
izes the characteristics of an idealized person. Empathy
is a form of identification in which the individual feels
the same *as* another person, rather than feeling *for* another person.

EXAMPLE: A young girl idealizes her home economics
teacher and decides to make the study and teaching of
home economics her career.

introjection—Introjection is similar to identification and
imitation, but introjection has a much greater effect on

31

the ego. The ego of the individual takes on another's ego and becomes like the other ego. The other person is internalized and incorporated into oneself.

EXAMPLE: The young child incorporates the personality of a significant adult and actually behaves like that adult.

projection—A denial of feelings and emotions that are unacceptable to one's self-image and attributing these characteristics to others comprise the mechanism of projection.

EXAMPLE: A student nurse states, "That patient doesn't like me." In reality the student's unconscious dislike of the patient is unacceptable.

rationalization—An individual who rationalizes makes acceptable excuses for behavior and feelings that are unacceptable to the self-image.

EXAMPLE: The nurse fails to give out medications on time and excuses feelings of inadequacy by stating, "There is just too much work and interference on this ward. No one could get things done on time."

reaction-formation—Reaction-formation is a mechanism by which a person unconsciously reverses true feelings, which are unacceptable to the self-image, and assumes the exact opposite behavior.

EXAMPLE: A mother who overprotects her child, not allowing any freedom at all, does so to make up for her unconscious feelings of rejection. She is not aware of these feelings and would vigorously deny their existence.

regression—Lack of satisfaction and threatened security occurring at any period of development can cause an individual to return to an earlier, more comfortable level of development. This is known as regression.

EXAMPLE: A person who has to smoke when under tension is reverting back to having needs met at the oral level.

repression—The involuntary exclusion from the conscious level of thought of those ideas, feelings, and situations that are unacceptable to one's self-concept is known as repression. This material is maintained at the unconscious level, where it continues to influence behavior. This influence is exhibited through blocking, slips of the tongue, and unrealistic fears.

EXAMPLE: A married woman who finds another man attractive involuntarily excludes this unacceptable feeling from her conscious level of thought and cannot understand why she continually forgets the gentleman's name.

sublimation—In sublimation socially acceptable behavior is substituted for unacceptable instincts because the expression of these instincts would prove a threat to the ego.

EXAMPLE: Unacceptable aggressive impulses gain social acceptance when utilized by the professional football player or boxer.

suppression—Suppression is the voluntary exclusion from the conscious level of thought of those ideas, feelings, and situations that produce discomfort and some anxiety. This material is maintained at the subconscious level and can be brought back to the conscious level without a great deal of effort.

EXAMPLE: A student who gets a poor report card "forgets" to give it to his parents for their signature.

transference—Emotional attitudes that were previously present toward important figures in the life of an individual are applied and attributed (transferred) to another person in the present.

EXAMPLE: An elderly female patient sees the nursing student as her granddaughter and responds to her in the same manner.

Study questions

1. Explain how defense mechanisms protect the ego.
2. Identify why defense mechanisms tend to develop during the formation of the superego.
3. Give three examples of how you have used specific defense mechanisms to control anxiety.
4. Explain why defense mechanisms are sometimes considered unhealthy.
5. Explain how a nurse may help a patient use defense mechanisms in a therapeutic manner.

CHAPTER 5

Communication

The drive to communicate is innate in all human beings. Just as the metabolic functions tie human beings to their physical surroundings, communication connects them to their social surroundings.

The purpose of communication is the transmission of emotions, ideas, and attitudes from one person to another; it is the means by which one mind may affect another. The term *communication* includes all forms of written and oral speech, music, pictorial arts, and the theater.

There are two components in communication, the verbal component and the nonverbal component. The more senses involved in the act of communicating, the more complete and accurate will be the message. When nonverbal perceptions and expressions do not function, verbal communication becomes difficult and sometimes impossible. For example, in communicating with someone face to face, one may receive the complete message, verbal and nonverbal, since all the senses are involved. In communicating by telephone, however, hearing is the only sense that is available. The nonverbal component is limited to the tone of the voice and the choice of the words. As the utilization of the other senses is impossible, a good deal of the message may be missed. In communicating by letter or note, the plain words on a piece of paper may result in most of the real message being missed. To understand the importance of the verbal and nonverbal components, imagine the senses being eliminated one at a time; this demonstrates how much can be missed if all the senses are not utilized.

Communication contains both conscious and unconscious

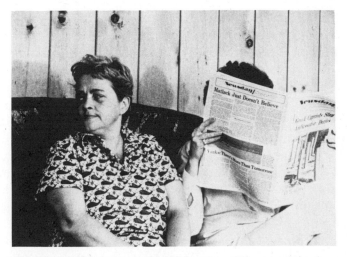

Fig. 4. Proximity does not always foster verbal communications.

material. Many of the thoughts and actions that have been repressed since childhood may be communicated unconsciously to a careful observer. Most of the nonverbal component is unconscious and offers the observer the opportunity to learn more about another person by being alert to these modes of expression.

Communication is not only observed but experienced. To be able to fully communicate, one must be able to perceive, interpret, and transmit. In today's computer world the inability to communicate effectively with the computer, which can neither perceive nor interpret, is creating additional problems in communication.

To be understood, a message must be phrased in terms that are understandable to others. Only when the receiver understands the message can the communication become meaningful. For example, very adequate directions transmitted in a foreign language cannot be considered as communication.

Since people need a certain amount of gratifying communication to learn, to grow, and to function in a group, all events that significantly curtail communication will eventually produce serious disturbances. Communication is the tool used by

35

individuals in their relationships with others. Interpersonal relationships can be defined as the actions and reactions between two people. The aim of one's action is to produce a reaction in another person. For example, if infants want to have their hunger satisfied, they soon learn that the behavior of crying will produce the desired reaction in their mothers.

The aim of interpersonal behavior may be conscious or unconscious. The individual may see others as they really are, or as someone else. They may communicate something in the present or something in the past. It must be emphasized that, unless the individual is conscious of the self and has an accurate picture of the other person, the interpersonal relationships will be distorted.

Difficulty in early interpersonal relationships elicits an immediate response and also leaves traces inside the person that will continue to exert an effect on the behavior. When interpersonal relationships become too frustrating, the individual finds ways to protect the self by withdrawing, screening, or otherwise controlling the relationship.

Patients come to the hospital with many past and present feelings and experiences that have influenced or will influence the present situation. They may be worried about their physical condition and have fears about the unknown, but their feelings for authority figures and other factors from the past may interfere with or inhibit their ability to relate with the hospital staff. Since all illness causes some degree of anxiety and regression, it can be assumed that the patient's interpersonal relationships will be distorted.

The primary goal of the interpersonal technique is to assist patients in reducing the distortions in interpersonal relationships. The nurse carries out this technique by helping patients identify their present problems and by assisting them in setting realistic goals. These goals can be accomplished if the nurse communicates a helping attitude to the patient. This desire is communicated by accepting patients as they are and by making them as comfortable as possible, so that anxiety will be lessened.

The most effective tools in interpersonal relationships are *listening* and *observing*. Animals in the jungle utilize hearing and sight far more effectively than humans do. The very appearance of humans (two ears, two eyes, and only one mouth) presents a clue as to how these organs should be used.

Study questions

1. Give an example of each of the three parts of communication.
2. Explain how interpersonal relations are affected by and affect communications.
3. Give at least five examples of nonverbal communication you have observed and identify what the person was attempting to communicate.
4. Identify at least ten factors in the hospital environment that can interfere with the patient's ability to perceive communication.
5. Identify at least five statements the nurse may use to assist patients to communicate and reduce their distorted views of reality.

Part two

THE RELATIONSHIP
BETWEEN PHYSICAL ILLNESS
AND EMOTIONAL PROBLEMS

Patients with emotional problems resulting from physical illness

Physical illness creates emotional problems for all patients. The behavior manifested during illness is the behavior the individual will demonstrate during any period of anxiety and is a defense utilized to control and limit this anxiety. The person who usually responds in a placid manner will probably become more placid, while the person who usually responds in a hysterical manner will usually become more hysterical. Although the previous personality and the ability to handle anxiety play a major role in an individual's reactions to illness, the situation in today's hospitals appears to contribute greatly to emotional problems. Patients are admitted to the hospital and immediately have most of their personal belongings and valuables removed. They are expected to adapt to and follow routines, with little explanation or reason given. They must accept a great deal on faith from the hospital staff, yet receive little in return for this faith. Many of their questions go unanswered, people enter and leave their rooms at will, and their personal identity is lost in the maze of the hospital environment.

The three psychic phases of illness

The three psychic phases of physical illness that the nurse will encounter are anger, depression, and denial. Individuals may show their anger in many ways. It may be turned inward

41

with increased physical symptoms or outward as explosive behavior toward anyone in the immediate environment. They are angry because they feel deserted. They have let themselves down. It is a time when the psyche is trying to battle the illness and all that it implies.

This is a time when the nurse needs to explain in detail all that is to be done for the patient. The nurse needs to take into consideration that the patient who is angry has a need to express this anger to a willing listener if the anxiety is to be reduced. The nurse can best help by giving the patient an opportunity to vent feelings without taking offense, for often this feeling of anger is falsely directed at the hospital personnel. The nurse can help the patient over this rough period by communicating an understanding that this is a very trying time and that the staff will be available to help. This is conveyed to the patient by realizing that the anger is not expressed against the staff or family but against being dependent. The nurse meets the patient's dependency needs in a matter-of-fact way while encouraging independent functioning. At this time the patient may be afraid to say, "I cannot do this myself." The nurse should take time to have the patient express feelings about any limitations. The nurse should never tell a patient not to worry, for that would be denying the patient the right to express true feelings about being ill. A statement such as, "You must feel poorly; tell me about it," is a better approach, as it gives the patient the opportunity to express feelings of anger to a willing listener. Communication with another person reduces the need to utilize more defensive behavior to maintain the ego.

If the patient is unable to express this anger, the psychic phase of depression may develop. The patient is now grieving over a loss, will look sad, may refuse to eat, sleeps poorly, and has problems with elimination. The behavior is no longer demanding and complaining, for at this stage the individual has pulled a cover around the self for protection and it is more difficult to make contact. The only time there is any expression at all may be when someone dear visits; the patient may then try to vent all previous anger on this visitor. This is a time when the nurse needs to help the family understand that the patient's grief is real and that some means of expressing this anger is

42

necessary. The nurse can help the patient express grief by conveying understanding and acceptance of these feelings. The nurse should never enter a room with a cheery "Hello" and a "My, how nice you look." Rather, the nurse should quietly sit with the patient even though there is no verbal communication. Remember, the patient is literally suffering from a psychic loss and has lost the battle to reduce anxiety. Quite often the nurse may be tempted to shock the patient out of this apathy, but this never works. Rather, by staying for longer periods and returning often, the nurse can convey a caring attitude that will help the patient through this experience.

If the depression is not resolved the patient may enter the psychic phase of denial, which is often seen in the chronically ill. Staff, family, and friends begin to feel as if the patient is emotionally and physically improved. The patient begins to show more interest in what is going on in the environment, but this interest is superficial and a cover for true feelings. Attention and interest are focused on minute detail rather than actual situations. The patient cannot become attached to any one person for any length of time, as there is a fear of being hurt. The patient may try to deny that there is actually a need for others or that there is physical illness. The nurse and the family may respond by not mentioning the illness at all. The patient may attempt to go home before being physically able or try to remain in the hospital much longer than necessary. When discharged, it may take a long time before the patient can actually feel close to the family again.

The patient's defenses must be supported, but there should be encouragement to verbally identify problems, for there cannot be a denial of illness in hopes that by some magic it will go away. The nurse can best help the patient and the family at this time by becoming involved. This is not easy. The patient who can look at you but not see you, who can talk but talks over you, who can hear but does not listen, needs a nurse who can accept this behavior and still want to help. The nurse can best assist this patient to relearn to trust others by assisting with the process of rehabilitation and self-acceptance. These goals can be achieved by developing a patient-centered plan for care in which the individual's desires are considered and there is a consistency of approach.

43

Acute and chronic brain disorders

Although all physical illness does create emotional problems, certain types of physical illness, such as the acute and chronic brain disorders, can produce profound emotional disturbances. Nurses employed in the general hospital may encounter patients with these disturbances in all wards and divisions.

ACUTE BRAIN DISORDERS

The acute brain disorders are caused by disturbances with circulation, infectious agents, metabolic factors, drug or alcoholic toxicity, and trauma. The emotional disturbance is usually caused by interference with the oxygen, nutrition, or fluid and electrolyte supply of the brain. The individual will go through four observable levels of behavior—confusion, delirium, stupor, and coma—if the physical interference is not corrected.

Confusion of the sensorium is usually the earliest symptom of brain disorders and is often the first clue that a problem exists. The patient is disoriented as to time and place and appears listless and lethargic. Restlessness and irritability occur with little provocation from the environment. As the physical interference with the brain cells progresses, the patient becomes increasingly more difficult to arouse and the confusion deepens.

As the level of delirium develops, the patient's behavior becomes more disorganized. Muscle coordination is poor, speech is slowed and slurred, and many thoughts are now controlled by the unconscious. Delusions, illusions, and hallucinations are common, and there may be a great deal of meaningless activity as thoughts and actions are no longer related. There is a gross disorientation of time, place, and person; these individuals do not know who they are, where they are, or what is happening. They are extremely frightened. Meaningful communication becomes difficult, if not impossible, as they progress toward unconsciousness.

If the physical condition continues, the patient will pass into a state of stupor and become extremely difficult to arouse.

44

This is a semiconscious state in which people and objects have little meaning. As the energy is now totally utilized in self-preservation, there is little or none left for emotional contact with the environment.

If the physical condition is not corrected, the patient will become comatose. At this stage there is no emotional contact with the environment. Response is possible only at the reflex level.

The nursing care for the patient with an acute brain syndrome has as its goal the alleviation of symptoms. If the temperature is high, immediate care should be instituted to bring the temperature down. If there is a lack of oxygen, it should be given. Drugs ordered to reduce infection should be carefully administered.

The problem of increased intracranial pressure is common; the nurse must remain alert to such symptoms as a slowing of pulse and respiration rate, a rise in temperature and blood pressure, an irregularity of the pupils, cyanosis of the nails and lips, and twitching or convulsive movements. The patient should be observed at very frequent intervals; if any of these symptoms are noted, they should be immediately reported to the physician.

The nurse can best help the patient with an acute brain syndrome by being competent in giving physical care. The nurse should strive to make the environment as safe as possible and can best accomplish this by keeping the patient under close observation. The patient needs someone to be there to give care and assurance. It does little good to try to teach at this time, for there is little contact with reality. Stimulation should be kept at a minimum, for rest is important. The nurse should not disagree with or try to talk the patient out of the delusions, illusions, or hallucinations but should accept the behavior as part of the illness. Reality is the theme the nurse can bring to the patient, but there should not be surprise or discouragement if the patient is not able to accept it. The nurse may not be able to make any sense out of the patient's rambling but should avoid antagonizing the patient by asking for clarification as this will only increase the anxiety, and anxiety will increase confusion.

CHRONIC BRAIN DISORDERS

The chronic brain disorders are associated with cerebro-vascular changes, toxic agents, tumors, congenital and genetic factors, and the residual effects of infectious agents and trauma. The behavior changes found in patients with chronic brain disorders are the results of permanent brain damage that exaggerated the previous personality.

Today, the number of patients with cerebrovascular changes is increasing because there are more aged people in our population. If the vascular changes cause a localized degeneration, the condition is classified as cerebral arteriosclerosis, while the diffuse degeneration of cells is classified as senility. Arteriosclerosis has a sudden onset and occurs in persons 40 to 50 years of age. The individual is very upset over the confusion and mental lapses. There is difficulty remembering the present but good retention of the past. The symptoms may lessen but they do recur and increase when the individual is under stress. This cycle tends to repeat itself until the person is no longer able to make adequate contact with reality. It is usually at this time that the patient (or the family) seeks hospitalization. Small cerebrovascular accidents are common; the early symptoms of headaches and confusion are frequently overlooked.

Senility has a much slower, gradual onset and occurs later in life, usually after 60 years of age. The individual seems to adapt to the degeneration as it occurs. The individual consciously makes up stories to fill in memory loss, and actions may seem odd. The individual can be maintained at home unless the behavior becomes unsafe or causes family conflict.

The nursing care for patients with cerebral arteriosclerosis is similar to that for patients with senility. The patient needs a protected environment where there is respect as a person and where independent strivings are supported and encouraged. The environment should remain fairly constant, but occasional changes of scenery are important so that contact with the outside world is maintained. Daily routines should be developed. The patient should be oriented to time, place, and personnel several times a day. Since the patient demonstrates frequent unprovoked changes in mood, the schedule of activities should remain flexible, for nursing care can be best administered when the patient is in a friendly and receptive mood. Dentures, glasses, and hearing aids should be used whenever necessary to aid in improving the declining senses. Good nutrition with vitamin supplementation may slow the pace of the brain cell degeneration, so particular emphasis should be placed on dietary needs. Eating can become more pleasant if familiar foods with a variety of flavors are served in smaller portions, with provisions for between-meal snacks. Proper exercise is vital, as joints tend to stiffen. A week in bed or in a wheelchair can change a fairly active person into an invalid. An hourly exercise schedule should be maintained, even if it is limited to walking only a few steps. When feasible, the patient should be encouraged to exercise the hands and arms by caring for physical needs such as hair combing, showering, and shaving.

The nurse should strive to assist the patient to maintain a self-identity. This can best be accomplished by encouraging the patient to wear personal clothing, adjusting the environment to better suit the needs, and respecting the rights of the individual. These steps will go a long way toward supporting the patient and preventing the rapid regression that often occurs when the patient is removed from the home environment.

Common interest groups may be formed spontaneously or may be planned by the staff. These group activities tend to enlarge the patient's social contacts, encourage abilities, and foster and maintain independence and self-reliance.

These patients frequently complain of physical symptoms as a means of seeking attention from the staff. However, medical causes for these complaints must be carefully ruled out before this assumption can be made. The nurse can help the patient avoid the necessity for these complaints by giving the attention required before it has to be sought in this manner. The patient needs someone to talk with, someone who will listen to the stories even when they are repeated over and over, someone who will not point out shortcomings but rather encourage and praise strengths.

The family of the elderly patient should be encouraged to make frequent visits and to take the patient home for short periods whenever possible. The patient's family may need to

47

be reminded that lapses in memory for the present and constant recall of the past are caused by illness and that their irritation will only create an increase in these symptoms.

GENERAL PARESIS

Another disease that clearly demonstrates the effects of central nervous system degeneration is general paresis. This disease is caused by an invasion of the brain cells by *Treponema pallidum,* the microorganism that causes syphilis. The patient may have become infected years earlier, with the acute symptoms going undiagnosed and untreated until the cerebral symptoms become apparent. There is a general muscle weakness, with fine muscle tremors, that may progress to paralysis. The speech is slowed, slurred, and confused. Writing is a difficult task, and penmanship is impossible to read. Skin rashes are fairly common, bone lesions are often present, and the pupils of the eyes no longer respond to light.

The behavioral symptoms are usually quite psychotic or neurotic. The personality appears to degenerate, with the defensive structure greatly altered by the illness. Common symptoms are rapid mood swings, irritability, restlessness, talkativeness, loss of appetite, and insomnia. The patient may be withdrawn, suspicious of others, and obsessed with grandiose ideas.

The nurse can best help the patient by support and prevention of further deterioration. Penicillin is given in large doses and can arrest the disease, but will not reverse the present level of brain damage. In caring for the patient in the hospital, the nurse should recognize that the behavior may become very aggressive at times, for the frustration tolerance is very low. Activities should be structured and limited to those that can be tolerated and enjoyed. These patients can be cared for and directed, once the nurse learns to deal with and accept their intolerance of others.

CHRONIC ALCOHOLIC DETERIORATION

Although toxic agents, such as drugs, and metabolic disorders may cause permanent brain damage, the nurse will most often care for patients with chronic alcoholic deterioration.

The patient with this condition usually has a history of heavy drinking, without proper nutrition, over a prolonged period. The first behavioral sign is usually a series of lapses in memory. The patient unconsciously attempts to compensate for these lapses by using confabulation (making up stores to fill in the gaps).

Physically the patient may demonstrate slight to severe tremors with some degree of neuritis. These symptoms result from a deficiency in vitamin B related not to the increased intake of alcohol but to the decreased intake of nutrients. Large doses of vitamin B are usually ordered for these patients to prevent further nerve irritations.

There is a gradual decline physically, emotionally, and socially. The patient loses contact with reality and the behavior becomes suspicious, impulsive, and uncontrollable. Social controls are no longer available, and many of the primary drives and wishes are acted out. The nurse can assist the patient by helping to reestablish the physical, emotional, and social standards that have been neglected. Physically, the nurse can provide the rest, exercise, and nutrition that is needed. Emotionally, care should be centered on the patient as a person with a drinking problem rather than as a drunk. A great deal of patience is required to communicate effectively with this patient, for there is a tendency to make up some words while juggling the meaning of others. For example, "frozen peas" may be used to communicate a feeling of coldness. Socially, the nurse can encourage the family to visit and can foster contact with other patients and the hospital staff. Even though the patient's behavior may be bizarre at times and limits must be set, a loss of contact with people and surroundings will only add to the confusion and regression.

Mental deficiency

Mental deficiency or mental retardation refers to a less than normal intelligence and is classified as either mild, moderate, or severe. If the lack of intelligence is mild, the person is educable and can be taught a vocation that does not require a great deal of abstract thought. There is some capability for simple reading, writing, and arithmetic. The individual frequently

49

takes a longer time to learn a task, but usually carries it out to the smallest detail once it has been learned. Such a person needs to be protected in dealings with society, for these individuals often become the prey of criminals and other deviates.

Individuals with a moderate lack of intelligence are trainable and can be taught to care for most of their activities of daily living, such as personal hygiene, bathing, dressing, elimination, eating, and exercise. They will usually be unable to read and write and have difficulty in learning any vocation. They frequently will require a sheltered environment for their own safety. They may be taught rote tasks, but the teaching is a long and trying experience.

The person with a severe lack of intelligence is untrainable and is totally dependent on the environment. Others have to provide complete physical, emotional, and social care. Usually these individuals require institutionalization, although some may be totally cared for in the home.

Although the cause of a high percentage of mental retardation is now known, there is always some guilt involved when a family learns that their child is retarded. The nurse can help the family by providing them with the opportunity to express and talk about their feelings. The nurse also assists the family by helping them plan and provide care for their child. This child will need more assistance, guidance, and support than the normal child if emotional problems are to be avoided. This care should provide for the development and maintenance of a self-identity, teaching based on the ability to learn, normal outlets for emotional drives, encouragement of independence whenever possible (both overprotection and underprotection should be avoided), and opportunities for enlargement of limited social competence. It is also extremely important that the parents or those caring for this child make some provisions for their own recreation, for relief from the constant supervision is essential.

The development of schools with teachers educated to care for these special children has opened new horizons. The parents should be encouraged to send their children to these schools and to become involved in the educational process.

50 When a mentally retarded person is hospitalized or institutionalized, the nurse must remember that the chronologic age will bear little relationship to the mental age and behavior. Individuals of 25 who have a mental age of 5 cannot be expected to fully comprehend reality or control all of their behavior. Their level of understanding has to be taken into consideration in planning and providing for physical and emotional care. The nurse can help maintain and, at times, improve the intelligence of the individual who is mentally retarded. People with a limited intelligence may improve or at least broaden their horizons while under the care of a nurse who gives them a chance to try, understands if they fail, and is truly excited about their success.

Study questions

1. Identify and describe the emotional support the nurse can provide the patient during the three psychic phases of physical illness.
2. What physical and emotional signs should clue the nurse that the patient's intracranial pressure has increased?
3. Describe the physical and emotional symptoms of arteriosclerosis and senility and identify their similarities and differences.
4. Taking into consideration the patient's physical, emotional, and social needs, identify the steps the nurse can take to provide a therapeutic environment for a patient with a chronic brain syndrome.
5. Prepare a schedule of activities that will provide for the emotional needs of patients at each level of mental retardation.

CHAPTER 7

Patients with physical illness resulting from emotional problems

The body that becomes ill as the result of emotional problems is said to be speaking an "organ language." Instead of finding healthy outlets for anxiety, individuals with psychosomatic illnesses seem to turn the anxiety inward on themselves. As they cannot verbally express anxiety, they seek to reduce and control it by expressing it through a particular organ. In these individuals anxiety appears to be a precipitating factor in the development of pathologic changes in reasonably healthy organs. The precise causes of psychosomatic disorders are unknown. Heredity and environment appear to play a role, but that role is uncertain. It is believed by some that emotional problems are coupled with a genetic weakness of a particular organ and that an irritation of that organ is manifested whenever anxiety is increased. Others believe that involvement of a particular organ results from a learned response to anxiety that has been passed through families for generations.

The person who develops a psychosomatic illness is thought never to have completely resolved the struggle of dependent needs versus independent strivings in childhood. The demands on the individual increase with growth, as do the fears of failure. Anxiety stimulates the autonomic nervous system; in these patients the nervous and endocrine impulses appear to center on one particular organ, resulting in signs and symptoms of irritation and illness. The illness seems to serve a twofold purpose for these patients. Because they are ill, they can focus their anxiety on the illness and they do not have to face the situation, which is really the basic problem. In addition, they derive secondary gains from the care and sympathy they receive from others. It is important to remember that the person with a psychosomatic illness is truly ill and is not faking to avoid an unpleasant task. There is a need for quality medical and nursing care during both the acute and chronic phases of the illness. Since the basic problem lies in the emotional area, this patient can often benefit from psychotherapy, which should be directed toward developing a more meaningful way of expressing anxiety.

Asthma

Asthma is a classic example of the psychosomatic illnesses affecting the respiratory tract. The cause may be allergic or psychic in nature but is most frequently a combination of both factors. The psychogenic basis is thought to date back to the threat of losing the mother's love. The child is dependent on the mother, and this fear of separation brings about a "cry for help." Since the child is also struggling and protesting against wanting this dependency, the "cry" is stifled and held back. The gasping during the asthmatic attack is thought to be symbolic of this stifled cry.

In caring for this patient the nurse should keep the relationship on a reality basis and as matter of fact as possible. The patient should be encouraged to talk about feelings rather than focusing on the physical illness. The nurse should be careful to avoid bringing into the situation any material that may stimulate the conflict in the patient's unconscious. The nurse must understand that any signs of overconcern may be seen as overprotection and may cause the old struggle between separation and helplessness to recur.

Peptic ulcer

Peptic ulcer is a psychosomatic illness that affects the upper gastrointestinal tract. The psychogenic basis is thought to date back to an early period in the formation of the personality. The child wants and needs to take in the mother's love and affection

53

but struggles against this need for dependency and expresses the desire for independence. As the child matures, competition and increased responsibilities add to the fears and anxiety. The child unconsciously longs to be loved and cared for, but these earlier feelings result in an outward striving for independence and success. These conflicting feelings create constant anxiety. The anxiety triggers the autonomic nervous system and results in an increased flow of hydrochloric acid. This high acidity irritates and finally ulcerates the mucous lining of the upper gastrointestinal tract.

The nurse can help by being a good listener and encouraging the patient to talk about feelings and conflicts while limiting the discussion of physical illness. Since the nurse recognizes that the patient has many unconscious dependent needs, the plan of care should include encouraging dependency during the acute stage of the illness. Only through a close interpersonal relationship can the patient work out these dependency needs and move toward independence with less fear and anxiety.

Ulcerative colitis

Ulcerative colitis is a psychosomatic illness affecting the lower gastrointestinal tract. The psychogenic basis is related to unresolved ambivalent feelings of love and hate. A person with ulcerative colitis demands love, and hates when it is not given. This individual cannot express either of these feelings outwardly and has a great deal of unconscious guilt about them. The anxiety level is high, and the individual tries to resolve and limit this anxiety and guilt by developing compulsive behavior such as an overconcern for orderliness and cleanliness. If the compulsive defenses do not succeed, ulcerative colitis may develop. The frequent explosive bowel movements are considered symbolic of the underlying hatred, while the tearful, pleading apologies for their odor and frequency are considered symbolic of the demand for love.

The nurse needs to be aware that the patient's strong ambivalent feelings may produce a superficial acceptance of all routines and treatments while they are actually being disregarded and rejected. The nurse should attempt to observe for compulsive behavior as a clue to the level of anxiety. The nurse

54

should not try to interfere with the compulsive actions but should focus on the anxiety causing the actions. This patient should be encouraged to express these angry feelings and real desires.

Essential hypertension

The person who has developed essential hypertension appears to be always on guard unless the defenses are broken down. The psychogenic basis is related to the fact that the individual has never learned to express inner feelings of hostility and aggression because of a fear of rejection and the need to be dependent. Outwardly the individual appears very self-controlled; although some hostility and aggression may be demonstrated, this is merely the overflow of what lies beneath. The individual needs prestige, status, and acceptance and literally seethes with anger when these needs are not met. The anger triggers the autonomic nervous system's "fight" mechanism and causes a constriction of the arteries and increased arterial pressure. Patients can often identify when their emotions are getting out of hand by the thumping sound in their head and increased heart rate.

The nurse can best assist these patients by helping them to express their hostility in an accepting atmosphere. If the nurse can accept and stay with them, they may learn that some hostility can be expressed without fear of retaliation or rejection.

Study questions
1. Describe the role of the autonomic nervous system in psychosomatic illness.
2. Identify the role played by heredity and environment in psychosomatic disorders.
3. Explain the statement, "The psychosomatic illness itself often increases the underlying emotional problems."
4. Psychosomatic illnesses are often believed to be "all in the mind." Explain why this is an incorrect statement.
5. List the activities the nurse can provide for the patient to help meet dependent and independent needs.

Part three

PATIENTS WITH EMOTIONAL DISORDERS

CHAPTER 8

Patients with psychoneurotic disorders

Unlike the person who has a psychosomatic disorder, the individual with a psychoneurotic disorder does not have a physical cause for the symptoms. The nurse will most likely care for these patients in a general hospital, although patients who are psychotic also have psychosomatic and psychoneurotic problems. A psychoneurotic disorder is thought to be the result of a conflict between internal and external stresses. The ego attempts to protect the personality against these stresses by developing such defenses as severe anxiety, depression, conversion, dissociation, phobias, obsessions, and compulsions. The patient who utilizes these defenses displays few defects in the ability to test reality and rarely responds with any severe antisocial behavior.

The nurse must keep in mind that the patient utilizing psychoneurotic defenses develops such symptoms to reduce the anxiety. Until the anxiety is lessened, the symptoms are needed and the nurse should not attempt to make the patient abandon them. Any pressures to change or modify behavior will create additional stress and anxiety for this patient and may well produce an increase in the psychoneurotic symptoms.

The medical treatments generally used for patients with psychoneurotic disorders include hypnosis and Sodium Amytal to uncover the basis for the symptoms, tranquilizers and energizers to alleviate the symptoms, and psychotherapy to interpret the underlying reasons for the problem and to assist

59

in reconstructing the personality to use healthier defenses.

In the late nineteenth and early twentieth centuries the most common types of psychoneurotic defenses were the conversion hysterias and the phobic reactions. The types of defenses appear to have changed since that time; today the population seems to be plagued with anxiety reactions and obsessive compulsive behaviors. The reason for this switch in choice of behavior is unknown but may have some relationship to changes in child-rearing practices and a weakening of sexual taboos.

Anxiety reactions

An anxiety reaction is characterized by the occurrence of a diffuse "free-floating" anxiety. There is a pervasive continuous tension and anticipation of danger. The onset of symptoms may be dramatic, usually occurs in late adolescence or early adulthood, and may begin with a choking sensation and trouble in swallowing. There is a fear of fainting, dying, and losing the mind. The patient is fidgety, worried, and cannot concentrate. There may be episodes of dyspnea, palpitations, tightness in the chest, weakness, headaches, increased cardiac and respiration rates, and tremors. The patient may complain of severe insomnia; however, it rarely interferes with usual activities. The symptoms seem to occur when the person feels insecure and is faced with either real or symbolic danger. The cause appears to be related to very early child-parent relationships, where the child learns the response either from the anxious overprotective parent or from an environment that has little structure and offers few guidelines for behavior.

A complete medical workup should be done to assure the patient that there are no physical causes for the complaints. The nurse cannot ignore the symptoms but must set limits on the verbal replay of them. If this is not done, nursing care can be lost in the physical complaints. Provisions must be made for adequate rest periods, and the patient should be encouraged to develop plans for a healthy balance between work and play. The anxiety of the environment should be kept to a minimum. The patient will feel less anxious if it is known beforehand what is to be done and what is to be expected.

Obsessive compulsive reactions

Obsessive compulsive reactions are marked by repetitive thoughts and actions that the person cannot change or stop. The patient is usually rigid, orderly, and perfectionistic. The individual tends to be miserly and stubborn and sets strict ethical and moral codes. Cleanliness and neatness are stressed and great attention is paid to minute details. Close relationships with people are avoided and an attempt is made to intellectualize all problems. There is usually a ritual involved with the compulsion, and the act is always accompanied by this ritual, which is used to ward off anxiety.

The onset usually occurs in adolescence or early adulthood but is usually related to problems that occurred during bowel training if there was too much stress or overgratification placed on the products of elimination. The conflicts of dependency versus independency are repressed and in later life are retriggered by anxiety-producing situations.

This is the most difficult type of psychoneurosis to treat, for the awareness of reality does not stop the obsessive compulsive behavior; the patient becomes tense and depressed if the compulsion cannot be carried out. Nursing care is limited to supporting the patient and providing an atmosphere of acceptance and understanding. It may be possible to reduce the patient's compulsions by limiting stress-producing situations in the environment. For example, patients who feel their hands will become dirty if they touch a doorknob should have their doors left open or should be provided with paper towels to turn the knobs.

Phobic reactions

Phobic reactions are characterized by overwhelming fears of particular objects or situations. Individuals utilizing these defenses learn to live with their fears by avoiding the particular object or situation. Phobias are common in children but may appear any time in life when the individual is under prolonged stress.

The basis for phobias dates back to the period when the individual was trying to work through the emotional problems with the parents. These individuals fear bodily harm and probably suffered a lack of love, security, and affection in their childhood. They crave love but cannot love or trust others, and they develop feelings of general unhappiness, resentment, anger, and hate. The anxiety about these feelings creates discomfort and interferes with their ability to function successfully. They unconsciously transfer their feelings of anxiety and hostility to a symbolic phobic object or situation. Once this is accomplished, they avoid the object; this reduces their anxiety and permits the development of a better relationship with others. If the phobias multiply, the person may require hospitalization, as it becomes impossible to avoid the phobic objects or situations and thereby reduce the anxiety.

The most common types of phobias are the following:

claustrophobia—the fear of being closed in

agoraphobia—the fear of open spaces

acrophobia—the fear of heights

zoophobia—the fear of animals

The chief nursing goals are the provision of companionship and the development of trust. The patient should never be forced to endure the phobic object or situation as a method of desensitization. This patient needs someone who can understand these fears and does not make light of them, someone who will stand by and try to reduce the stresses in the environment. It is in this trusting relationship that the patient may open up and talk about these deep feelings.

Conversion reactions

Conversion reactions are characterized by a sudden impairment of motor or sensory functions without an organic reason for the symptom. The classic feature of this psychoneurosis is the patient's almost total indifference and lack of anxiety about the illness. It should be recognized that the patient has transferred the anxiety to a symbolic physical ailment and has therefore reduced emotional pressure. The symptoms are utilized for primary and secondary gains. The primary gains are the saving of face and the removal of a stressful situation. The secondary gain is obtained when the family and others feel sorry for the patient and try to meet any physical needs. The symptoms usually develop during adulthood but have their basis in the child-parent relationship; the patient has never resolved the guilt and fears created by feelings of love for the parent of the opposite sex and feelings of hostility toward the parent of the same sex. The patient's history will frequently show a stressful childhood and the occurrence of frequent accidents and illnesses.

Nursing care should be aimed at supporting the patient's need for the symptoms and the development of a positive relationship. Stress in the environment should be kept to a minimum. Again, as in other psychoneuroses, the nurse should understand that the symptoms are real to the patient and serve as a defense against anxiety. The nurse does not try to tear down these defenses but becomes the eyes for the patient who cannot see and helps with the chores of daily living for the patient who cannot move.

Depressive and dissociative reactions

Two other types of psychoneurotic disorders are the depressive and dissociative reactions. Many of the symptoms that are seen in the psychotic patient are also seen in patients with these two types of psychoneurotic reactions. There is one main difference: this patient remains in contact with reality and the total personality is less disturbed. The primary impulses of the id have not been able to forge themselves into the total personality because of the depressive or dissociative defenses.

The patient with a depressive reaction looks and acts sad and has an overwhelming feeling of worthlessness. The depressive reaction frequently follows some situation that would usually cause some depression; however, this depression is deeper and more prolonged. The depression may also be precipitated by a threatened failure or an increase in responsibility. There is no suicidal ideation or avoidance of functions, as seen in the psychotic depression. The patient can work and assume responsibility but derives little pleasure from any activity. Usually the onset of symptoms is gradual. The whole syndrome of grieving is taking place. The patient looks and feels depressed because life has not lived up to expectations. There is anger at the world, but, since this anger cannot be accepted or expressed, strong feelings of guilt arise. The anger is turned in-

63

ward and the guilt is expressed in the form of grief. Life has lost its spark. These symptoms may be observed to some degree in all ill patients, but for the psychoneurotic patient they are not very easy to work through. The basis for this type of defense goes back to very early childhood when there was total dependence. The patient again wants to be dependent, but this desire creates anger. The feelings of guilt reappear, and anxiety increases and is expressed through the depression. Individuals using the depressive defenses almost seem to seek opportunities to experience a loss or be proved a failure.

In caring for the patient who has a depressive reaction, the nurse should try to meet these dependency needs. There will be times when the patient may not feel like doing any daily care; the nurse should administer the necessary care in a matter-of-fact way without increasing the patient's anxiety. The nurse should not try to talk the patient out of the depression. Remember, the depression is a defense and trying to talk the patient out of it will only deepen it. These individuals need an understanding mother-substitute who can help them to express their feelings outwardly rather than turning them inward. An available nurse may go a long way in helping these patients learn to limit expectations without the need for guilt or anger.

The dissociative reactions are characterized by the individual's attempt to deal with anxiety by walling off certain areas of reality and escaping from the stressful situation. The defensive mechanism utilized is repression. Such an individual is essentially very immature and has a great inability to handle anxiety. The types of dissociative reactions include amnesia, short flights from reality known as *fugue states,* sleepwalking, and the unusual multiple personality. The true dissociative reaction is extremely rare, and the nurse will seldom have the opportunity to care for patients with this diagnosis. These patients need a great deal of support to assist them in coping with the stress they are experiencing.

Study questions

1. Describe the problems in childhood that may develop into each type of psychoneurosis.
2. Explain how the use of psychoneurotic defenses limits the individual physically, emotionally, and socially.

3. How do the patient's complaints and the nurse's observations differ for individuals with psychoneurotic and psychosomatic problems?
4. What nursing approach can be universally beneficial for all patients with psychoneurotic problems?
5. What type of activity is most beneficial for patients with psychoneurotic problems?

CHAPTER 9

Patients with personality disorders

Personality disturbances are regarded as borderline states falling somewhere between the neuroses and the psychoses or somewhere between ordinary conduct and deviant behavior. Personality disorders are regarded as chronic and are deeply ingrained in what might be called the character or essence of the individual. The personality, instead of utilizing symptoms expressed in mental, somatic, or emotional terms in its efforts to secure adjustment, uses patterns of peculiar actions or misbehavior. The personality disorders are characterized by defects in the development of the personality or by pathologic trends in its structure. Individuals with these disorders have little if any subjective anxiety about their behavior and are without the distress often observed in other types of emotional problems.

The personality disturbances are divided into three main groupings: personality pattern disturbances, personality trait disturbances, and sociopathic personality disturbances.

Personality pattern disturbances and personality trait disturbances

The personality pattern disturbances include the inadequate, the schizoid, the cyclothymic, and the paranoid personalities. The symptoms of these disturbances are very similar in nature to the psychoses. The individuals lack the flexibility necessary for maximum social adjustment, but they are usually able to adapt minimally and thereby avoid the necessity for hospitalized psychiatric care.

The personality trait disturbances include the passive aggressive, the emotionally unstable, and the compulsive personalities. The symptoms of these disturbances are usually not as profound or incapacitating as those presented by patients with the personality pattern disturbances. Individuals in this group are characterized by an inability to maintain their emotional equilibrium when under stress. When not under stress they are able to make a fairly good, though superficial, adjustment. They rarely require psychiatric care unless placed under severe stress for prolonged periods. These individuals rarely require psychiatric hospitalization.

The nurse will usually care for patients with personality pattern and trait disturbances in a general hospital where these patients have been admitted for unrelated physical reasons. The nurse provides an atmosphere where patients feel accepted as they are, meeting not only physical needs but many of the patients' emotional and social needs as well. The person who is superficial and withdrawn, has mood swings, or blames others is difficult to cope with. If the nurse remembers that these patterns of behavior are long-standing and have little relationship to the immediate situation, the focus will be on the patient as a person rather than on the behavior. Nurses must recognize and face their true feelings about the patient, for if there are negative feelings that are interfering with their ability to approach the patient therapeutically, someone else should care for the patient.

Sociopathic personality disturbances

The sociopathic personality disorders include the dissocial reactions and the antisocial reactions. The sociopathic personality is characterized by the feeling that whatever is done is all right. Persons with a sociopathic disorder may break every law, steal, cheat, lie, even murder and have absolutely no guilt or sorrow for their actions. They can be master "con men" and have an uncanny skill in convincing others to believe in them, although they cannot be trusted. There appears to be a total lack of superego or moral conscience control, and the person-

67

ality seems completely self-centered. The basis is thought to rest in the failure of the parents to meet very many of their early emotional needs. Some of these individuals have been shown little love or kindness by the parents and have never learned how to show these traits to others. Still others have been overindulged by the parents and never learned the give and take necessary for successful interpersonal relationships. They are insensitive to the needs and feelings of others and have not learned how to relate in a friendly, helpful manner. As a result of these factors, these individuals are cold, self-centered, and distrustful. Some actively and aggressively behave as if they wished to take revenge on someone for the deficiencies in their own early lives. Others misbehave more passively and in subtle ways seem to expect society to understand, accept, and ignore their deficiencies.

Individuals with sociopathic personality disorders are very difficult to treat. They usually do not want or seek help, are usually not hospitalized, and frequently find themselves at odds with the law, spending time in penal institutions. Psychiatry has made some inroads lately, especially with those patients who have some motivation to change. The therapy is directed toward the reconstruction of the personality. The atmosphere is very strict and the staff takes a stern attitude and will give approval only to that behavior that is considered socially acceptable. These patients have to learn how to treat others, and such learning is difficult this late in life. Many psychiatrists believe that these patients have utilized their acting out as a defense against their basic insecurity. They successfully prevent anyone from getting close to them and so protect themselves from being hurt. Once these patients can truly express their feelings, they may be able to give up some of their antisocial defenses.

The nursing care for these patients must be focused on reality. The nurse should exercise care and avoid being taken in by their charm. They will always attempt to be in control of the situation and will manipulate anyone to achieve this control. If it serves their purpose, they will attempt to cause a chasm between the doctor and nurse or between the nurse and another patient. The entire staff must agree on the approach to be used and the limits to be set for these patients, for consistency is vital. The nurse is the authority figure, an authority figure who will listen and accept suggestions but who also sets limits.

Study questions

1. Discuss why individuals with personality disorders have little subjective anxiety.
2. Recall some of the patients for whom you have cared and list the personality trait disturbances observed in them.
3. Explain why the personality pattern disturbance is more incapacitating than the personality trait disturbance.
4. What part of the personality is incomplete or underdeveloped in the sociopath and what is the probable cause for this deficit?
5. What activities would be most helpful to assist the individual with a personality disorder?

CHAPTER 10

Patients with addictive disorders

People who depend on drugs, alcohol, or any combination of drugs and alcohol to decrease their anxiety are considered to have an addictive personality disturbance. Such individuals have difficulty in tolerating stress, are unable to handle anxiety on a mature level, and reach for these outside crutches to maintain themselves. The drug or alcohol supplies the boost they need, for it blurs reality and makes it more tolerable. The price for their addictive maintenance of the ego is high, for they soon cannot feel whole without the drug or alcohol. Gradually they replace social, emotional, physical, and financial drives with the bottle or pill. It is the demands they make on others that usually bring them into conflict with society.

Drug addicts cannot be satisfied with their previous "fix," for they develop a tolerance and constantly need an increased amount of the drug to maintain their physical and emotional equilibrium. The development of tolerance is a physiologic phenomenon that requires addicts to take what would ordinarily be a lethal dose to satisfy their needs. For unknown reasons, this tolerance may disappear without warning and the previous tolerable dose becomes an overdose, often resulting in death. Some habits cost hundreds of dollars a day to support. To maintain their habits, individuals turn to antisocial behavior such as prostitution, shoplifting, and other criminal acts to get the money to buy the drug. They then become deviates, not only on the interpersonal level, but in society at large.

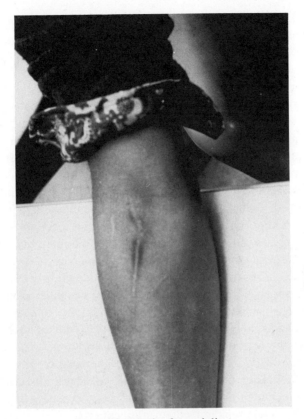

Fig. 5. The track of a mainliner.

Alcoholics are usually able to maintain their habit within the laws of society. Alcohol may be purchased in most states. If the cost of the bottle is not earned, it is usually obtained by begging from family, friends, or strangers, or by the sale of personal belongings. The alcoholic's conflicts are usually with the family or employer.

The alcoholic or drug addict has replaced family, friends, and society with a habit, a habit that is necessary to increase internalized feelings of worth. Both the alcoholic and drug addict may make repeated vows to give up their habits, but few have the ability to succeed without help. Perhaps one can understand how difficult this really is by recognizing what they are being asked to give up. It is their total protection, their total

71

reality, their unfailing friend who helps them appear bigger in their own eyes. In addition, when off their habit, they may have periods of guilt. The guilt produces more anxiety and increases the need for the habit.

In caring for patients with addictive personalities, nurses must examine their own feelings about this behavior. No other group can arouse such hostile feelings simply because they are so weak. As one nurse put it, "It's not that *I* don't care about their problem, it's just that *they* don't." The family and friends feel as if these individuals have not only let themselves down but have let those who care down as well. The nurse frequently shares their feelings. Society expects each individual to be able to live within the confines of the moral and legal code. Any action against this code will usually have a double reverberation—personal guilt and society's condemnation.

The basis of the addictive disorders is thought to be feelings of inferiority. These patients have strong dependency needs, which are usually unmet. Outwardly they may appear easygoing and friendly, but inwardly they seethe with an anger that they cannot express. Their anger has been internalized. They show the world that they do not care, when in fact they care a great deal. They feel guilty about their feelings and seek relief in alcohol and/or drugs. They have difficulty in setting limits for themselves and seek immediate gratification for their needs and immediate relief from discomfort.

The most effective approach in helping addicted individuals appears to be through groups. Addicts seem to learn from people like themselves to whom they can talk about their faults without their world crumbling around them. People with the same problems seem able to give the best support. They can point out when individuals are trying to fool themselves and others, for this is better accepted from a peer group.

Alcoholics Anonymous and Narcotics Anonymous are nonprofessional groups composed of ex-addicts. The individual who receives the most help from these groups is that individual who wants to be helped. Many persons attend meetings because of the pressure of family and friends, but only the addict is capable of kicking the habit and to be successful they must find other means of bolstering their ego.

Methadone maintenance programs have proved to be of some help for the long-term, hard-core addict. It must be recognized that these programs simply transfer the addiction from illegal drugs to a legal one. However, the long-term addict may be able to return to an acceptable level of functioning in society with a minimal amount of the drug. Methadone has been shown to produce problems in the newborn and should not be given during pregnancy.

With the increased use of addictive substances, the nurse needs to be aware of the more commonly used drugs, the symptoms of use, and the signs of withdrawal. The nurse should become familiar with the list on pp. 74-75 and report any findings when they are observed.

In caring for addicted patients, the nurse must be equally concerned about their physical, emotional, and social needs. Physically patients may be in dire need of good nutrition, vitamin supplements, and a planned schedule of exercise and sleep, as these are the areas most often abused and neglected by these patients. Close observation during the detoxification phase of treatment is essential because of the increased incidence of problems resulting from mixed addictions to a variety of drugs or to drugs and alcohol. The nurse should carefully explain the hospital procedure and regulations to the patient, family, and friends. No drugs or alcohol are to be brought in from outside the hospital. Nurses should not try to act as police but should be concerned with setting the tone for the structured environment and understanding that the patient is going through a rough time. The nurse should support the patient but should not tolerate any nonsense. Addicts will try to test the controls, and the nurse should identify this behavior to them. By remaining consistent the nurse can help patients learn to accept these outside controls until they are able to develop their own. Reality needs to be pointed out, as these patients frequently try to manipulate and distort it. Psychotherapy is directed toward helping the patient reconstruct the personality, by helping to identify and work through the problems. Group therapy gives the patient the opportunity to try out new defenses in a structured fashion.

The patient should be encouraged to become involved with

73

community groups where time can be spent in helping other addicted individuals to help themselves. This type of involvement helps the patient meet some of the dependency needs, fosters independence, and bolsters self-image.

DEPENDENCY DRUGS

Drug	Symptoms	Withdrawal
Opiates— morphine, heroin, methadone (synthetic opiate)	Nodding and sleepiness Reduction in activity Flushing, itching Constriction of pupils	Nervousness Yawning, watery eyes and nose Dilation of pupils Severe ache in back and legs Increased respirations and elevated temperature Vomiting, diarrhea Abdominal cramps
Depressants— sedatives, barbiturates	Slurred speech Staggering gait Sluggish reaction Erratic emotion	Nervousness, headache Muscle twitching Weakness, insomnia Tremors, convulsions Decreased blood pressure
Stimulants— cocaine, amphetamine	Excitability Talkativeness Feeling of euphoria Dilation of pupils Increased blood pressure	Mental depression Fatigue
Alcohol	Smell of alcohol Slurred speech Staggering gait Loss of sphincter control Delirium Unconsciousness	Delirium tremors Muscle twitching Convulsions Disorientation

NONDEPENDENCY DRUGS*

Drug	Symptoms
Hallucinogens — marihuana, LSD	Euphoria, exaltation Dreamy, floating state Enlarged pupils Disturbed, distorted senses Suspension of time LSD may produce a bad trip where extreme panic, fear, and general psychotic behavior may appear
Solvents — glue, hairspray, freezone, gasoline	Blurred vision, confusion Staggering, slurred speech May affect circulation, kidneys, liver, and central nervous system

*No true dependency, but may lead to the use of dependency drugs.

Study questions

1. Describe the basic personality problem of the individual with an addictive disorder.
2. Explain why addiction creates physical and social as well as emotional problems.
3. List other addictive substances in addition to narcotics, barbiturates, and alcohol.
4. What nursing actions can assist the patient during the detoxification phase?
5. What activities would be most beneficial to the addictive patient during the rehabilitation phase?

Part four

PATIENTS WITH FUNCTIONAL PSYCHOTIC ILLNESSES

CHAPTER 11

Tools utilized in psychiatric nursing

The nurse is becoming more and more involved in preventing emotional illness and caring for patients after hospitalization as part of the mental health team. In prevention, the nurse should be aware of the crisis periods in a person's life, when emotional stress may be increased. Illness, the stages of growth and development, and the real or imaginary losses that occur in a lifetime can all create a serious strain on a vulnerable personality.

Individuals need intervention during a crisis because their problem-solving responses are inadequate to handle the additional stress. Before the crisis the individual apparently functioned at some level, but the rise in tension results in a stage of upset that causes ineffectual behavior. The individual attempts to mobilize the defenses by seeking new ways of attacking the crisis. This may include hopeless resignation or perceptual distortion of the crisis in an attempt to relieve the discomfort. If the problem continues despite attempts at reorganization, the individual may experience a major disorganization of the personality. The outcome of this disorganization depends on the precrisis physical and emotional status of the individual, the perceptions of the present situation, and the external resources available to assist during the crisis period.

During crisis the support group can help the individual to problem solve by being well-organized, having a system of authority that is clear and acceptable, keeping the lines of communication open, and supporting the individual's decisions in handling the problem. During the rise in tension the nurse should support and aid by encouraging the use of tension-releasing defenses. The individual's personality sets the perimeters, but the outcome is determined by the interplay of internal and external forces. The individual who wants help and seeks it is more likely to receive it.

To support an individual during a crisis the nurse should:

1. Create an atmosphere that will help the individual feel free to discuss problems.
2. Be receptive and willing to listen to the individual's concept of the problem.
3. Listen closely for the description of symptoms rather than a superficial discussion of the problem.
4. Start where the individuals are, help them recognize where they are, and demonstrate an understanding of their feelings.
5. Focus on how the individual feels about what is happening.
6. Accept the fact that the individual may have a need to distort reality if problems are unbearable and focusing on it or giving false reassurance will not help.
7. Focus the individual by asking specific questions such as:
   a. What is the length and onset of the problem?
   b. What efforts have been made to cope with the problem?
   c. What help has been previously sought?
   d. What has occurred since then?
8. Observe the individual's behavior, watching for optimistic or pessimistic attitudes.
9. Help the individual avoid dependency by encouraging thoughts about alternate solutions.
10. Develop an objective, collaborative relationship that focuses on the individual's feelings rather than content.

Any exaggeration or changes in an individual's behavior, such as rapid mood swings, loss of sleep and appetite, irritability, physical complaints, withdrawal, attacking or blaming others, should be recognized as early signs that the person needs help. The nurse can create an environment in which anxiety is lessened but needs to report any symptoms to the physician so the patient can have immediate medical help.

The stay in a psychiatric hospital should be limited to care during the crisis period, and provisions for early return to the community should be included in the plan of care. Many general hospitals now have an acute psychiatric care unit so that the transition from the community to the hospital and back into the community is made easier. Most patients are encouraged to seek voluntary admission to a psychiatric hospital, and commitment by the doctor or the courts is becoming the exception rather than the rule. Once patients are admitted, their mental status should be frequently reviewed and a concentrated effort should be made by all involved in their care to help them return to the community as soon as possible, for it has been demonstrated that prolonged hospitalization adds to the deterioration of the personality.

All hospitals should include facilities for treating the emotional problems of people in the community. These facilities ideally include outpatient clinics, day and night care centers,

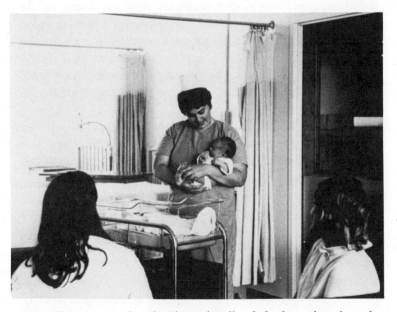

Fig. 6. The nurse teaches the "know-how" to help the patient through periods of crisis.

halfway houses, and home-care services. The nurse assigned to the clinic along with the psychiatrist, psychologist, and social worker has the opportunity to help patients talk about the problems they are experiencing in the community. In addition, the nurse may have the opportunity to observe them and to be with them during treatments and group sessions. In the day- and night-care centers the nurse provides the therapeutic environment for patients who may be spending only part of their time within the hospital and the rest of their time within the community. Home-care services provide for continuity of care by following up patients in the community. Here the nurse observes and helps patients in their own environment. The community is becoming increasingly involved in helping people to help themselves recover from the impact of emotional illness. The nurse must realize that most patients can become contributing members in the community and can handle their anxieties if some provision is made to assist them during periods of crisis.

Nursing has a unique and essential contribution to make to individuals with emotional problems who are living in the community. The primary focus of community nursing is on those daily living activities that are causing problems for the individual and the family. In observing these daily living activities, the nurse becomes aware of the interrelationship between the psychological problems and the environmental situation.

Community psychiatric nurses make their contribution to the psychiatric team as a social psychiatric model. There is a tremendous need for this type of nursing care because the traditional method of treating individuals in psychiatric inpatient facilities does not prepare them for life outside the hospital. As psychiatric patients move into the community, the emphasis must shift from the hospital to the external environment to meet the patients' current needs.

In community psychiatry the nurse becomes involved in the social environment of the individual. This means that nursing is no longer caring on a limited scale but is looking at society through the eyes of the individual. The nurse becomes involved in the whole social environment of the individual. This may range from rehabilitation, to vocational training, to living arrangements.

In community psychiatry the major emphasis is on the group process and the use of groups within the environment as therapeutic tools and educational therapies. The emphasis throughout is focused on the individual's strengths and developing methods for problem solving.

The preferred locale for treatment is in the home or the community itself. The focus should be on the present, dealing with specific problems in the vocational, marital, or physical areas and specific behavioral changes that are needed. Nurses can use their surrogate image to help individuals with the realities of everyday living. The most appropriate approach is through physical contact, socializing activities, and informal interviews.

The main problem area for most individuals seems to be in the area of developing organizational patterns so that they will make better use of themselves in relationship to their society. The second major problem is one of dependency. Years of seeing the world as hostile and not allowing oneself to express wants and needs creates a false dependency on others.

The community nurse works with the family and tries to help them understand the behavior of the individual and find satisfactory solutions to the problems of daily living. The nurse assists the family by helping them to organize the household and divide its responsibilities among its members, including the patient. The community nurse also assists members in good nutritional shopping, meal planning, budgeting, personal hygiene, and health care.

Community psychiatric nurses should be knowledgeable about somatic therapies and the relationship between the social, physical, and mental disorders. They have been given the responsibility of ensuring discharged psychiatric patients that they will receive coordinated and continuous services from the hospital to the community—a community that will accept them because the community psychiatric nurse is there.

Although the material in this chapter pertains to psychiatric nursing situations in general, it is more specific for patients with functional psychotic illnesses such as those in Chapters 12

83

and 13. The student should refer back to Chapter 6 for the specific nursing approaches for patients with organic psychotic illnesses.

Guidelines for psychiatric nursing

The following guidelines for psychiatric nursing can and should be utilized by nurses in all patient situations.

1. Nurses should recognize their own feelings and how these feelings affect their behavior and relationships. Nurses must recognize that all behavior has meaning to the person performing the action and that some anxiety is basic to all human activity.

EXAMPLE: Miss Donald, the nurse, hears that Mr. James, the patient to whom she has been assigned, does not want her as his nurse. She starts toward his room with feelings of anger. Then she recognizes that these feelings of anger will only increase the patient's anxiety. Miss Donald thinks of Mr. James and how anxious he must be to say he did not need a nurse. When she was thinking of herself, she had heard the patient did not want her as his nurse. When she thought of Mr. James, she understood he was too anxious to want *any* nurse.

2. The nurse must accept and respect the patient as a person, regardless of behavior. The nurse may at times reject or ignore a patient's behavior without rejecting the patient. Patients must be given the opportunity to use those defenses they need to use.

EXAMPLE: The patient yells at the nurse, "Go away, I don't need you, you are all monsters." The nurse responds, "You must be very upset. Let's talk about it." The nurse has helped the patient by not focusing on the behavior. The nurse recognized the patient as a person with feelings, and it is the person with feelings that becomes the focus.

3. The relationship should be a therapeutic one. This means that the nurse has to focus on how patients feel about themselves and their lives. Any discussion of personal problems should be initiated by the patient. The nurse should center on the patient, not on the control of the symptoms. The nurse's objectivity is a therapeutic tool.

EXAMPLE: The patient states, "It's this lousy hospital. No one ever tells me anything. I'm just a freak." The nurse responds, "You feel you are being treated differently. . . ." The patient agrees, saying, "That's it, everyone comes in and pokes at me without saying a word." The nurse says, "I can understand your feelings." The patient responds, "It always makes me angry when someone looks over me." The problem was initiated by the patient. The nurse focused on the patient's feelings, not the symptoms, by using an objective approach.

4. The first aim of the nurse-patient relationship is for the nurse to reduce the fears and anxieties of the patient. The nurse encourages the patient to express both positive and negative feelings and accepts these feelings rather than giving false reassurance.

EXAMPLE: A patient states, "Why is it everytime I get sick I feel so helpless?" The nurse responds, "Could you explain this feeling?" The patient says, "It's as if all my rights have been denied. People tell me when to go to sleep, wake up, eat, and exercise, even when I have visitors." The nurse answers, "This makes you feel like you're not in control of the situation. . . ." The patient, "Yes, I feel I'm treated as a baby." The nurse, "Tell me more about this feeling." The nurse supports the patient without giving false reassurance and reduces fears and anxieties by encouraging the expression of feelings.

5. The nurse must accept and meet the dependency needs of the patient while fostering and supporting attempts at independency. The nurse recognizes that the nonverbal rather than the verbal communications are more expressive of the patient's true feelings. Patients may interpret their own behavior, the nurse should not.

EXAMPLE: A young male patient becomes quite upset and tearful while talking with the nurse. He states, "I'm a young person; men don't cry but I'm afraid I'm going to become a burden to my wife. I have always been the strong one. My wife is not too well either." The nurse responds, "I can understand why you feel like crying. I'll stay with you until you are feeling better." A period of silence follows, the

85

patient continues to cry but tries to control his emotions. The nurse states, "It must be difficult for you." The patient, now sobbing, responds, "No one knows what I have been through, I feel so useless." The nurse says, "You are going through a very rough time." The nurse does not interpret the patient's behavior but rather reflects the feeling tones recognized in his communication. The nurse attempts to meet his dependency needs by supporting his independence.

6. The nurse must help patients set appropriate limits for themselves. When they are out of control, they are asking for control. The nurse should present reality to them while conveying an understanding of their feelings.

EXAMPLE: A patient turns to the nurse and says, "The doctor said I am to get out of bed, but I'm a cripple and cripples can't walk." The nurse replies, "I know this is not going to be easy, but I will help you. We will take it very easy; if you feel any discomfort you can rest. When would be the best time for you to get up?" The nurse has helped the patient by understanding and accepting feelings. The nurse presents the reality that the patient must get out of bed but allows the patient to help determine the limits.

7. The nurse must keep in mind that all patients have a potential for growth toward mental health. The nurse should also recognize that patients frequently meet the expectations of staff members. By expecting mentally healthy rather than mentally ill behavior, the nurse can help restore the patient's self-image.

EXAMPLE: The nurse enters the patient's room with a warm, friendly approach. She says, "My name is Miss Brown, I'm going to take care of you today." The patient replies, "I'm Mr. Jones, I need to have some fresh drinking water." The nurse gets him fresh water and then proceeds to help the patient plan for his care. She then gives care when he needs assistance and encourages him in activities that he can accomplish. When she leaves his room he smiles and says, "I feel like a different person." The nurse was surprised to learn from the staff that Mr. Jones was a "problem patient" who refused to do anything for himself. Miss Brown went into his room expecting the patient to respond appropriately, and the patient lived up to her expectations.

Therapeutic approaches in the nurse-patient relationship

1. The nurse should make the environment as therapeutic as possible—warm colors, home-like environment, and a furniture arrangement that encourages interpersonal relationships.
2. The nurse needs to understand the patients' feelings. The nurse recognizes that people use their defenses to protect themselves from anxiety. The nurse can best help reduce these defenses by helping them reduce their anxiety.
3. When talking with the patient, the nurse spends most of the time listening, is nonjudgmental in attitude, and reflects feelings rather than words.
4. The nurse meets patients on their own level. The nurse is truthful, always keeps promises, and is consistent in actions and attitudes.
5. The nurse acts to meet the patient's needs. The nurse explains everything to the patient and is flexible in planning routines and activities.
6. The nurse respects the patient's feelings and protects the patient's right to privacy.
7. When the patient's behavior is disturbing, the nurse rejects the behavior but never rejects the patient. The nurse limits the patient's behavior by using distraction and by offering indirect suggestions.
8. The patient is more comfortable and secure when informed of the limits that have been set. The patient may try to test these limits but they should remain firm. The nurse should give the patient as much freedom as can be handled, while helping the patient understand that certain controls are necessary to ensure individual safety and the safety and comfort of the entire group.

Common errors in interpersonal techniques

1. The nurse may be too authoritarian.
2. The nurse may fail to recognize that the nurse's behavior and presence are upsetting the patient and increasing anxiety.

3. The nurse may probe and focus on fact rather than feelings. Questions such as "Why?" put the patient on the defensive.
4. The nurse may try to talk the patients out of their feelings or symptoms or speak to them in a condescending manner.
5. The nurse may become sensitive to the patient's verbal attack and may try to defend personal actions or make excuses.
6. The nurse may fail to provide the strengths the patient is seeking by demonstrating personal insecurity and fears.
7. The nurse may think the patient is only pretending or faking and that behavior could be controlled if the patient wanted to control it. The nurse may also consider mental illness as a punishment for sin.
8. The nurse may forget that the patient is involved with the family and that the family is involved with the patient. The nurse may consider the family intruders, resent their questions, or blame them for the patient's problems.

Study questions

1. Describe what is meant by a therapeutic relationship.
2. Identify the steps you would take to help patients set limits on their behavior.
3. Identify the role and activities of all members of the mental health team.
4. Try to recall a nurse-patient relationship in which you have been involved. What were your feelings and how did your feelings affect the relationship?
5. Identify the facilities available in your community to prevent and treat emotional problems.

CHAPTER 12

Patients with schizophrenic reactions

It has been said that the neurotic person builds castles while the psychotic person lives in them; however, true psychosis is difficult to define. Behavior that is termed psychotic in one society may be accepted as normal in another. A vegetarian would be considered sick in a tribe of primitive cannibals, while a sadistic murderer would be considered sick in a civilized population. So it is the society that decides what behavior is or is not to be classified as psychotic. The presence of what may be termed psychotic behavior does not always result in the individual receiving treatment or being hospitalized, for other factors enter into the situation. A family may accept or make excuses for one of its member's behavior and never seek help or assistance. An entire neighborhood may accept and consider as eccentric that behavior observed in a familiar figure, while they may term the same behavior psychotic if it were to be observed in a stranger. Until recently neither the family nor society took the necessary action to force the psychotic individual into treatment unless the behavior impinged on or broke the moral, social, or esthetic values and codes of the society. However, the emphasis on mental health and mental illness during the last two decades has made the population more aware of the problems, and earlier help and assistance are now being sought for these individuals.

Childhood schizophrenia

The main psychotic illness occurring in young children is classified as childhood schizophrenia. This disorder is characterized by a pattern of deep withdrawal into oneself and a severe disturbance in personality development. This is usually accompanied by some physical, emotional, and intellectual failure. These symptoms can appear in varying degrees and create problems that can range anywhere from a relatively mild adjustment difficulty to a profound pattern of withdrawal from reality.

Although a great deal has been written about the faulty mother-child relationships as a factor in schizophrenia, many psychiatrists now believe that such a child responds differently from other children. The child's different response apparently creates increased anxiety in the mother, and her increased anxiety is transmitted back to the child; the child responds by withdrawing and exhibiting further indifference to the mother. Thus a vicious cycle in mother-child relationships is set in motion.

These children fail to learn to relate to others in a meaningful way, and since they derive little satisfaction from people, they begin to treat others as inanimate objects. They are autistic, live in their own world, and utilize an individualistic manner of thought and speech. They have a poorly developed ego and will rarely use the personal pronouns "I" and "me." They will typically refer to themselves by name—"Tom wants it" rather than "I want it." They may spend a great deal of time rocking and carrying out other very basic repetitive movements from which they apparently derive some pleasure and satisfaction. They are lonely, lost children who look past people to a dream world of their own.

Although such children are difficult to reach in psychotherapy because of their underdeveloped ego defenses and limitations in communication skills, a great deal has been accomplished by placing them in a small group where individualized attention can be given and firm, consistent, but realistic limits can be set. They desperately need one person who by establishing an atmosphere of warmth, comfort, acceptance, trust, and security can lead them from their dream world into the world of reality. The families of these children should be encouraged to express their feelings to an understanding staff member. They need a great deal of support, acceptance, and guidance and frequently derive great benefits from psychotherapy.

Schizophrenic reactions

Schizophrenic reactions occur most commonly in the teens and early twenties, although they may occur at any time in the life span when the individual is faced with overwhelming stress and anxiety. The incidence of schizophrenia is rather high in our society (approximately 1% of the general population), and it has been estimated that over half of all the hospital beds in the United States are occupied by patients with this diagnosis.

The cause of schizophrenia is not known at the present time. The biologist believes it is caused by genetic or physical factors, the psychologist believes it is caused by emotional factors, and the sociologist believes it is caused by sociologic factors. The person who develops schizophrenia does have some metabolic changes that seem to stimulate both social and emotional problems. However, whether these changes cause the schizophrenia or whether the schizophrenia causes the changes is uncertain. There does appear to be some disturbance in the family relationships of most of these patients. There is usually a history of a relatively cold, unstructured family life, where little emotional response was received from either parent. The child seems to develop a pattern whereby a withdrawal into self and away from others occurs. Although this self-investment helps the child maintain security, it creates a very unsatisfactory interpersonal life with little gratification obtained from relationships with others.

Persons with schizophrenic reactions demonstrate a lack of unification in their personalities and are unable to function as well-integrated individuals. There is a lack of meaningful interpersonal relationships and a decrease in intellectual functioning. They make foolish errors, are extremely gullible and naive, and have severe difficulty in forming new ideas. They demonstrate a reduction in motivation, will, and energy and are unable to establish or work toward a goal. In addition to these general symptoms, five other primary symptoms are related to these reactions, sometimes referred to as the "5 A's" of schizophrenia.

91

1. *Association*. These individuals have a great deal of difficulty in thought processes because of a disturbance in associative links. They cannot filter out unrelated, accidental thoughts, are easily sidetracked, become too specific about irrelevant things, and in general demonstrate a deprivation of logical thought.

2. *Affect*. These individuals demonstrate apathy, shallowness and blunting of emotions, and an inappropriateness of mood. They may look sad or happy, yet they emit no real feeling of sadness or joy. They have difficulty in enjoying pleasure and, as their affect lags behind their thoughts, they may laugh 1 or 2 minutes after others. Their moods may be grossly inappropriate—they may laugh at such things as funerals or they may cry on happy occasions.

3. *Ambivalence*. These individuals experience the occurrence of opposing ideas in all areas of their being. At the same time they may want to do and yet not want to do a specific act. They may know something is real, true, and valid and at the same time feel it is unreal, false, and invalid. They may love and hate the same object at the same time.

4. *Autism*. These individuals are rather detached from reality, for they live in a world where their inner fantasy dominates and excludes external reality. They are preoccupied with thoughts of function in life and find it almost impossible to relate to others.

5. *Attention*. These individuals demonstrate an interference in their ability to concentrate. This is a primary interference and should not be confused with the disruption in concentration that may be secondary to boredom or anxiety. These individuals may wish to learn, but their inability to concentrate hinders and prevents their learning.

Some secondary symptoms that may be seen in schizophrenia, as well as in other functional and organic psychoses, include hallucinations, delusions, memory disturbances, body image disturbances, and changes in speech and writing. These secondary symptoms are more disturbing to both the patient and the family and frequently precipitate the patient's seeking treatment.

In addition to an overlapping of many of these symptoms,

individuals with schizophrenic reactions may demonstrate those symptoms usually associated with the psychoneurotic, psychosomatic, or personality disturbances. These patients' ego boundaries have collapsed, and they are living in the frightening world of their own imagination. All of their symptoms are manifestations of their psyche's last stand to reduce the overwhelming anxiety they are experiencing.

Schizophrenic reactions occur in both acute and chronic forms. In the acute form the onset of the psychotic symptoms is usually rather sudden, there can be an identifiable precipitating stress, and the episode usually lasts for only a short time. In the chronic form the onset of the psychotic symptoms is usually slow and insidious, for the individual may exhibit what may be termed prepsychotic behavior many years before the defenses fail and the patient enters the chronic psychotic state.

The patient in the acute episode is easier to treat; in fact, it is estimated that fully 25% of these individuals will have a remission of psychotic symptoms with no treatment at all. It is

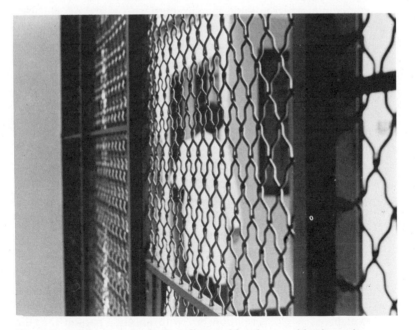

Fig. 7. Perception can be further distorted by the psychiatric setting.   **93**

important, however, that once treatment is started, it not be stopped because the psychotic symptoms have disappeared. If the underlying reasons for the behavior are not resolved, the symptoms will return, and each recurrent episode leads the patient toward the more regressive chronic form.

Nursing care

The nurse on the psychiatric service will care for many patients with the broad general diagnosis of schizophrenia. As this broad diagnosis only points to the primary symptoms the patient may be experiencing, a further classification according to general behavior has been used. This classification includes simple, catatonic, paranoid, hebephrenic, and undifferentiated types of schizophrenia. Over the years it has been recognized that few patients present the classic symptoms associated with any one particular type but rather present an overlapping of symptoms common to all types. The recognition of this overlapping has led to the increased use of the undifferentiated classification.

Simple schizophrenia is characterized by a slow, chronic, insidious poverty of ideas. There are few of the secondary symptoms, little or no anxiety, and very little fantasy life. These individuals are usually considered misfits in society. They demonstrate a lack of interest in any accomplishment, they want to be left alone, and they become irritated when forced into action. These individuals are seldom hospitalized and tend to become the tramps, vagrants, migrant workers, and prostitutes of society.

In caring for patients who lack interest in any accomplishment, the nurse must have a great deal of patience. Limits must be set, but these limits should be the same for all the patients on the ward. These individuals need to be treated as sick people not as malingerers; since they do not appear as overtly psychotic as other patients, unrealistic expectations are frequently set for them. When they are first admitted to the hospital, they should be gradually oriented to the routines, simple instructions should be given, and all rules should be thoroughly explained. A close relationship with another person may be frightening at first and may even create an increase in symptoms, but the nurse should use every effort to put them at ease. The nurse may have to set limits in relation to their activities of daily living, especially the areas of grooming, bathing, and dressing. Patients should be encouraged to participate in activities, but the activities should be meaningful and not frustrating. They must be helped to develop new ways of coping with anxiety and must learn to structure their behavior.

Catatonic schizophrenia is characterized by the utilization of rather unpredictable motor activity as a defense against anxiety. This motor activity has two extremes—one is total and utter inactivity and is referred to as the "stupor" or waxy flexibility state, and the other is wild, extreme overactivity and is referred to as the "agitated" or "fugue" state. A number of secondary symptoms are usually present—especially common are delusional thoughts and auditory and visual hallucinations.

In the stuporous, inactive state, patients remove their will from their actions and become immobilized. They are extremely suggestible, and when they do move it is in an automaton-like manner. They may resist any passive form of motion and may assume one posture for hours, days, or weeks. They may refuse all food and often lose control of elimination. They may imitate others or repeat exactly what others have said. They may be completely mute and appear totally disoriented and completely unaware of any activity occurring around them. It should be noted, however, that these patients are aware of much that is being said and done to them, even though they give no external clues to this awareness. It is not unusual for these patients to come out of this phase and repeat word for word the conversation they have overheard.

Nursing care during this phase is aimed at supporting these patients while attempting to keep the environment as anxiety free as possible. Nutrition must be maintained, and if spoon-feeding does not work, tube feeding must be initiated. The nurse should explain in simple terms everything that is being done to these patients, even though they may give no outward response. These patients need a nurse who will stay with them, protect and provide for them, and yet not demand responses from them. The mere fact that the nurse stays may help them

95

develop some feelings of worth, since these patients are truly in need of rebuilding their self-image.

Suddenly, without warning and without external cause, these patients may come out of this stupor and enter into the agitated, overactive, fugue state. Since they are responding to internal rather than external stimulation, they present extreme problems in nursing care. They need to be protected from harming themselves or others as their impulsive behavior makes them extremely unpredictable. For safety, they should be removed from the group into a secluded area and, if their behavior permits, someone should stay with them. It is important that the reason for this seclusion be explained to them, for they should not be made to feel they are being punished or rejected.

The nursing care for these individuals is difficult, for they must be protected from themselves. Their nutritional needs are increased by their overactivity, yet they frequently present severe eating problems and may have to be force-fed. They must be prevented from becoming exhausted; sedatives or tranquilizers may be necessary. They are desperately in need of support, understanding, and acceptance. Their resistance must be overcome if they are to receive this type of care.

Paranoid schizophrenia is characterized by a well-developed delusional system accompanied by somatic and auditory hallucinations. The delusions and hallucinations are usually persecutory in nature and extremely frightening to the patient. The paranoid type of schizophrenia occurs later in life, at about 30 to 35 years of age, and usually these individuals are better able to cover up their emotional regression than other persons with schizophrenia. On the surface their delusions of persecution may seem well-founded and logical, and it is not until the original basis for the delusion is uncovered that the psychotic origin of the thought becomes clear. They are irritable and withdrawn and frequently use many antisocial means to keep people away from them. They are usually fearful of others and try to keep people at a distance. They feel that the best defense is an offense, and so they verbally attack others without cause. They experience ideas of reference and believe that everything spoken or written by others, either in the newspaper, on television, or in any conversation, relates to them. They frequently develop delusions of grandeur and believe they are someone else, usually someone of importance. Early in life they learned to defend themselves from anxiety by the use of the projective pattern of behavior, and they continue to utilize this defense in their psychotic state. They blame others for everything that has happened to them, often focusing on people with power.

In caring for patients with paranoid schizophrenia, the nurse should recognize that they have unconsciously changed their world because reality was unbearable for them. The nurse should not point out the inconsistencies of their delusions but should try to reduce their anxiety so they will not need to use these psychotic defenses. These patients truly believe that people cannot be trusted, and the nurse must, by actions, attempt to disprove these feelings. The nurse should maintain reality for them yet should accept their need to deny it. Reality cannot be forced on these patients; if the nurse attempts to convince them they are wrong, it will only succeed in increasing their anxiety. These patients are extremely concerned with people watching and staring at them. The nurse should be aware that these patients need some eye contact but should avoid staring at them. They may nonverbally challenge the nurse to outstare them, but this challenge should not be accepted. These patients may react sexually toward the nurse; this may be an attempt to offend and keep staff members at a distance. If this is attempted, the nurse should calmly tell them that their behavior is not acceptable and that they will be left alone to regain control. These patients need someone in their environment who does not lose control, but who can maintain it in a calm, acceptable manner.

Hebephrenic schizophrenia is characterized by a severe regression, accompanied by a rapid deterioration in the intellectual and emotional processes. The behavior is usually extremely infantile, inappropriate, and illogical. The patient frequently utilizes bizarre mannerisms, giggly silly laughter, and self-coined words. The patient is delusional and disoriented and actively responds to both visual and auditory hallucinations.

In caring for patients with hebephrenic schizophrenia, the

97

nurse must protect them from their outer and inner environments. The inner environment can be made less stressful if the nurse is available to talk with these patients and get them interested in the outside world. If the pressures of reality are reduced, they will have less need to live in their inner world of voices and visions. The nurse should accept their bizarre behavior but should let them know that it is impossible to understand what they are trying to say. These patients may engage in childish sexual behavior such as masturbation, and limits should be set on this acting out. However, since these patients are easily distracted, the substitution of a simple task usually serves to halt the sexual behavior. The nurse needs to help them come out of their isolation and mix with other people. Some of the most severe hebephrenic patients have been helped to overcome their regression by a nurse who did not shun them, but who kept coming back. Perhaps the nurse's actions told them more than words ever could—that they were liked and were worthy of being liked as people.

As stated earlier, schizophrenia can occur at any time in the life of an individual when the anxiety and stress of living reach an overwhelming state. Some psychoses thought to be separate entities are now being considered as schizophrenic reactions; one of the more common of these is the postpartum psychosis. It is now generally accepted that the stress and anxiety associated with pregnancy, labor, and delivery may serve to produce an acute schizophrenic reaction soon after the birth of the infant. These patients respond well to treatment and frequently, with the help of psychotherapy, have no further psychotic episodes.

The nurse should be aware of the major medical treatments for patients with schizophrenia. The advent of tranquilizing drugs has helped make the patient more amenable to therapy and more manageable on the ward, but it must be remembered that these drugs cover the symptoms and do not remove them. Psychotic patients need to learn how to react and to control their reactions with people. Interpersonal skills can be learned by these individuals only when they have people to relate to, people who are concerned and actively involved.

Psychosurgery, wet packs, and other somatic therapies

were all utilized to control and limit the patient's symptoms before the tranquilizers came into use. Since the 1950s, however, the tranquilizers combined with psychotherapy, motivation, occupational therapies, and increased community involvement have been the treatments of choice. It is vital that the nurse in caring for patients who are being given tranquilizers remember that large doses are typically ordered for psychiatric patients and that observation for reactions or toxic effects is an extremely important part of nursing care.

The tranquilizers are divided into major and minor categories with the major tranquilizers, the phenothiazines, being the most commonly used in psychiatry. Examples of the phenothiazines include: Compazine (prochlorperazine dimaleate), Stelazine (trifluoperazine), Vesprin (triflupromazine hydrochloride), Thorazine (chloropromazine hydrochloride), Sparine (promazine hydrochloride), and Mellaril (thioridazine hydrochloride). Most tranquilizers are supplied in tablet, liquid, or intramuscular forms. The nurse should carefully observe the patient to make sure the medication has been swallowed. If there is doubt, the doctor should be consulted about changing the form of the medication. The side effects from these drugs include restlessness, sedation, seizures, impotency, dermatitis, chewing, grimacing, jaw protrusion, rocking, and pacing. These side effects can usually be controlled by reducing the dose of the tranquilizer or giving another medication to counteract the symptoms.

Laboratory work should be done frequently for all patients receiving tranquilizers, and the nurse should observe the patients carefully and report and record any signs of toxicity. These include decreased white cell count, which may produce symptoms such as sore throat or lesions in the mouth, and liver damage, which may produce jaundice. These toxic effects require that the drug be discontinued. The nurse should be aware of these symptoms and should report them if they are observed. It is sometimes difficult to determine whether these symptoms are the result of a physical illness or the result of the medication, but the doctor should make this decision.

In administering an intramuscular injection to a psychiatric patient, the nurse may need some assistance in holding the **99** patient. The patient should be encouraged to accept the injection, but if this cannot be accomplished enough assistance must be available to ensure that the injection is given as safely and quickly as possible. The longer it takes to administer the injection, the more anxious the patient becomes. The procedure should be explained, the arms and legs supported, and the medication given all in a matter of minutes.

The minor tranquilizing drugs are frequently administered to patients in the general hospital to reduce anxiety and tension. This category includes Equanil (meprobamate), Librium (chlordiazepoxide hydrochloride), and Valium (diazepam). Sedation is the most common side effect noted, and often these drugs are administered to increase the effectiveness of a sedative. Some other side effects include tremors, gastrointestinal upsets, and hypersensitivity, but these reactions are not usually severe. Some allergic reactions have occurred, but they usually appear at the beginning of therapy and most often clear up rapidly when the drug is stopped.

Some hospitals may still use insulin coma therapy in the treatment of patients with schizophrenia, and the nurse may have to care for a patient receiving this form of therapy. Since the patient will lose consciousness, loose clothing should be worn, false dentures removed, and breakfast withheld. The patient is in therapy practically all morning and, when returning to the unit, should be encouraged to shower and dress before eating a combined breakfast and lunch. For the remainder of the day it is the nurse's responsibility to carefully observe the patient for symptoms of insulin shock. These symptoms include nervousness, profuse perspiration and weakness, flushed or pale skin, and anxiety. If the patient exhibits any of these symptoms, orange juice should be given immediately and the doctor notified. If treatment is not given, the patient may become delirious, have seizures, and enter a comatose state; death can result. The dangers inherent in this therapy have resulted in its diminished use.

Electroconvulsive therapy is also used in the treatment of patients with schizophrenia. Both insulin and electroconvulsive treatments seem to make the patient more receptive to psychotherapy and interpersonal therapy, but how they do this

or why they do this is really not known. Since electroconvulsive therapy seems more effective in the treatment of patients
with affective reactions, it will be discussed in the next chapter.

Study questions

1. Identify why childhood schizophrenia is so difficult to treat.
2. List the five general symptoms that are considered classic for
   schizophrenia and give an example of each symptom.
3. What side effects occur most commonly with the major tranquilizers and for what symptoms should the nurse be alert?
4. List the signs and symptoms of insulin shock and identify the
   nursing care required when they occur.
5. What nursing approach would be most therapeutic for a patient
   using the withdrawn and projective patterns of behavior?

CHAPTER 13

Patients with affective reactions

The behavior of an individual with an affective reaction is characterized by disturbances in mood, emotions, and affect. The affective reaction psychosis can occur any time in the life span as a reaction to stress and anxiety when individuals who have tended to utilize the aggressive patterns of behavior turn their hostility and aggression inward on themselves. The three psychotic disorders classified as affective reactions include psychotic depressive reactions, manic depressive psychosis, and involutional psychosis or melancholia.

Psychotic depressive reactions

If a severe depression follows a precipitating factor in an individual over 20 years of age and if there is no history of previous episodes of depression or hyperactive behavior, the diagnosis of psychotic depressive reaction is usually made. Although this patient may demonstrate a gross misinterpretation of reality as a result of the illness, the prepsychotic personality is usually fairly stable and responds rapidly to a sound treatment program. As the nursing needs and medical management are similar for patients with any of the affective reactions, the care will be discussed later in this chapter.

Manic depressive psychosis

If repeated episodes of severe depression or hyperactive behavior occur in an individual between 20 and 40 years of age and if these individuals have been in control of their emotions and in contact with reality between these episodes, a diagnosis of manic depressive psychosis is usually made. A further

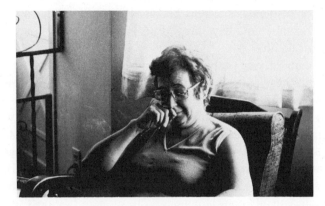

Fig. 8. The face of depression.

classification of this psychosis is based on the behavior presently exhibited by the patient and the history of previous episodes. If the patient is severely depressed and has a history of episodes of severe depression, the classification depressed type is added. If the patient is hyperactive, is demonstrating manic behavior, and has a history of episodes of this behavior, the classification manic type is added. If the patient is either severely depressed or hyperactive and has a history of episodes of the opposite behavior, the classification mixed type is added.

The onset of the depression is usually fairly rapid, and a predisposing factor is not always obvious to the outsider but is usually interpreted by the patient as a threat to security. These patients are depressed both physically and psychologically. They will demonstrate a severe dejection in mood, a slow-up of thought and speech, and a marked decrease in psychomotor activity. Insomnia, a decrease in appetite, a difficulty in performing daily tasks, and a decreased sex drive are usually present. These patients are logical and oriented, and rarely do hallucinations occur. They have an extremely low self-concept, feel worthless, and usually will speak about having "committed the unpardonable sin," which they never identify. They talk a great deal about suicide, but frequently during the acute stage their psychomotor depression is severe enough to prevent their carrying out their wish to die. As the depression lifts, the pre- **103** vention of suicidal attempts becomes an even greater nursing need, for they now have the physical energy to carry out their wish for death.

The underlying problem in the manic phase is also a depression, but these patients unconsciously deny they are depressed and overcompensate by acting opposite to what they feel. Instead of being depressed and withdrawing from contact with others, they race headlong into activity. They sleep and rest for only short periods, are constantly moving, monopolize all conversations, and are continuously planning and scheming. They appear to be in good humor but become rapidly irritable if their characteristically poor judgment is questioned. It almost seems that these patients are afraid that, if they stop for a minute, their depression will catch up with them and all will be lost. This extreme hyperactivity uses a tremendous amount of energy, and these patients must be protected from total physical exhaustion.

The prognosis for the patient with a manic depressive psychosis is good even without therapy and excellent with the therapy now available. Recovery is fairly rapid, and the patient may function for years before another episode develops.

Involutional psychosis or melancholia

If a severe depression occurs for the first time between 40 and 60 years of age and is associated with the menopause or climacterium, it is usually diagnosed as involutional psychosis or melancholia. The onset of symptoms is gradual, and the patient complains of insomnia, increased nervousness, agitation, fearfulness, and a severe melancholia. These patients have many somatic delusions such as feeling they are constipated and their bodies are rotting away. They are usually obsessed with fears of death and with delusions concerning sin and poverty. This disorder tends to occur in those individuals who demonstrate a rigid, inflexible, unadapting, overassertive, overly meticulous, and worrisome prepsychotic personality. Frequently, a precipitating factor such as the marriage of a child, the death of a loved one, or financial reverses can be found in their history. Although the mental ability of these patients is decreased by the depression, their motor activity is

104

increased. They are depressed, but their depression is an agitated depression, and they spend most of their time wringing their hands and pacing the floor. The threat of suicide is present throughout this illness, but these patients do respond fairly rapidly to treatment.

Nursing care

The nursing care of patients with affective reactions must have as its main objective the prevention of suicide, which is a very real threat throughout both the depressed and manic phases. There are between twenty and twenty-five thousand deaths from suicide per year in the United States, and studies have shown that better than two-thirds of these people communicated their intentions to someone before they acted. It is the nurse's role to recognize this communication and intervene before suicide is attempted. Frequently the suicide will occur as the patient's depression is lifting. The patient may state "I feel better and have worked things out." The nurse should not reduce her observations, for what the patient has worked out may be the decision and method of suicide.

The nurse can lessen the danger of suicide by removing from the environment all glass, sharp objects, belts, and shoelaces. The family should be instructed to bring pants with an elastic waist and slip-on shoes. At times it may be necessary to keep the patient under constant observation for 24-hour periods. Although this one-to-one observation ties up a nursing staff member for each shift, it does serve a dual purpose for the patient. First, it prevents the patient from carrying out the suicidal intentions; second, it communicates a feeling of worth to the patient that the staff cares enough to prevent the act. Since most patients with affective reactions have extremely low self-concepts and are rather overwhelmed by feelings of guilt, this communication of worth can assist in rebuilding the patient's ego.

Feeding problems are very common in both the depressed and the hyperactive phases and careful observation and recording of intake is vital. The depressed patient may feel unworthy of food, and the hyperactive patient may just not take the time to sit down and eat. Small feedings served at frequent

105

intervals, in a matter-of-fact manner, tend to be better received than large feedings on a set schedule. The staff should attempt to provide the hyperactive patient with food that can be carried by hand and eaten during activities. As the hyperactive patient is expending a great deal of energy during this constant movement, a high-calorie, high-protein diet should be provided. Rest periods should be encouraged, and sedation may be necessary to ensure that adequate rest is achieved. Because of the depression and hyperactivity, the nurse may have to provide these patients with almost all of their physical care and should keep a close check on their physical conditions.

Activities for the patient with an affective reaction should be of a simple, uncomplicated nature and should contain a great deal of repetitive material. These activities should be of short duration and should require little concentration. The patient should be helped to express anger and hostility in a manner that will not increase guilt. This can sometimes be accomplished by the use of a punching bag or some similar equipment. To get the depressed patient to become involved with any activity at all is a difficult task. Some of the patient's guilt can be relieved by doing menial tasks such as scrubbing the floor or washing the bathroom; the staff members should allow the patient to do these tasks. The therapeutic purpose of such tasks should be thoroughly explained to the family, as they can become very upset if they find the patient engaged in such activities.

Medical therapy is directed toward relieving the symptoms presented by the patient. Electroconvulsive therapy (sometimes called electric shock therapy) has been and continues to be very effective in the treatment of both the depressed and hyperactive patient. This treatment is believed to result in a breaking up of behavior patterns by creating a temporary amnesia. This temporary amnesia seems to help the patient forget the full emotional impact of recent events. When the patient's memory returns 3 to 4 weeks after the series of treatments is concluded, much of the self-deprecating, self-defeating affect is lost and can be replaced, with the help of therapy, by a more self-respecting, self-accepting attitude.

106 In preparing patients for electroconvulsive therapy, the nurse should remain with them and assure them that a staff member will be there when they awaken after the treatment. They may need to talk about their fears of the treatment or their feelings that they are receiving the treatment as a punishment, and the nurse should just listen and not try to interfere or interrupt their verbalization of feelings. Remember, these patients have a need for self-punishment and the nurse attempting to talk them out of these feelings may only succeed in making them feel more guilty. The patient should have nothing by mouth prior to the treatment, and all dentures should be removed. This is necessary since the electroconvulsive therapy will cause the patient to lose consciousness, and aspiration pneumonia must be prevented.

Following therapy, the patient will be disoriented and have difficulty remembering what has occurred; this memory loss increases with each treatment. The patient is often confused and, as a result, is usually frightened. The nurse should orient the patient, repeatedly if necessary, and explain what is causing the confusion. By staying with the patient and helping during this trying period, a close working relationship between the patient and the nurse can develop. The nurse should observe, report, and record the patient's response to the treatments.

In the treatment of manic depressive psychosis, lithium carbonate has clearly become the drug of choice. Because there are many adverse reactions to lithium and because toxicity can occur at close to therapeutic serum levels, careful observation and monitoring is necessary. The nurse must be certain that sodium depletion does not occur through situations such as the use of diuretics or dietary restriction of sodium or excessive sodium loss through sweating or diarrhea. The nurse should also observe the patient for severe tremors and symptoms of neuromuscular irritability, which indicates toxicity. Other medications often ordered for patients with affective reactions are tranquilizers, antidepressants, and mood elevators. The patient in the hyperactive stage frequently receives a combination of tranquilizers (discussed in Chapter 12) and antidepressants. There are two types of antidepressants, the shorter-acting noncumulative type and the longer-acting cumulative type.

The major short-acting antidepressants used today are the drugs Tofranil (imipramine hydrochloride) and Elavil (amitriptyline hydrochloride). These drugs do not increase the effects of sedatives or tranquilizers and may therefore be used in combination with such drugs. Elavil is also used in helping to arrive at a diagnosis; it will sedate a nondepressed patient, while it relieves a depression without sedating the depressed patient.

The longer-acting, more toxic antidepressants include Nardil (phenelzine) and Parnate (tranylcypromine). These drugs do have a cumulative effect and tend to increase the action of other drugs such as narcotics, barbiturates, sedatives, tranquilizers, antihistamines, antirheumatic compounds, antihypertensive drugs, and steroids. Because of this action, a patient receiving this type of drug should be instructed not to take any medication without the doctor's permission.

The side effects of the antidepressants include dryness of the mouth, gastrointestinal upsets, decreased appetite, headaches, increased perspiration, tremors, impotency, edema, nightmares, insomnia, confusion, and euphoria. In caring for patients receiving these drugs, the nurse should be aware of these side effects and report any symptoms or changes in behavior to the doctor as soon as they are noticed.

Study questions

1. Compare the differences between manic depressive psychosis and involutional psychosis.
2. What side effects occur most commonly with the antidepressants and for what symptoms should the nurse be alert?
3. How should the nurse respond when the patient says, "I'm going to kill myself"?
4. Identify the nursing care for a patient both before and after electroconvulsive therapy.
5. What activities would be most therapeutic during the depressed and manic phases of manic depressive psychosis?

CHAPTER 14

Remotivating the emotionally disturbed patient through groups

Remotivation is the urge to get moving again. *Social re-motivation* is a term frequently heard today concerning psychiatric hospitals. The social and psychologic elements of hospital living are being strengthened through a better understanding of group relations, better coordination of the resources of the entire hospital, and bridging the gap between the hospital and the community.

The hospital is a planned setting that should be as much like the outside community as possible. Support is needed in rebuilding the patient's ego functions, and the hospital group experience should furnish an atmosphere in which this can be accomplished. The patients soon understand that to be members of this hospital community requires that certain privileges and obligations be subjugated to group demands. Patients must learn to relate to two distinct groups—the patient group in which sibling-type relationships develop and the staff group in which authoritarian or parental-type relationships develop.

The nurse should be concerned with studying the individual in group situations to better understand how to plan, create, and use the therapeutic relationship. It is the social climate of a therapeutic environment that stimulates, motivates, and helps restore injured egos.

All patients bring to a group their own subjective experiences and ideologic choices. These two factors have to be **109** counterbalanced to achieve a realistic self-identity rather than continue the identity diffusion.

Everyone needs a group for protection, security, emotional needs, and identification. In groups individuals can see their self-images mirrored in others. The group begins to control the behavior of its members by accepting or rejecting their actions. As group membership brings satisfaction and support while providing intellectual stimuli and emotional outlets, the members strive for acceptance. By belonging to a group the patient is not alone, there are significant others with whom to identify. The rules of the game are set by the group and are ultimately accepted and internalized by its members. Group therapy is based on the fact that the patients' behavior is changed by belonging to and sharing with a peer group.

The three types of groups the nurse most often becomes involved with include:

1. *Didactic teaching groups*—the nurse attempts to give some information to the members in areas such as hygiene, dating, or dressing for a job interview. Ideally the members should have common interests, and the group should be small enough to encourage involvement of all present.

2. *Task-centered groups*—the nurse attempts to assist members to use problem-solving techniques to accomplish specific tasks. This type of group is usually most effective for planning activities, unit meetings, or any situation in which decisions involving group assignments are to be made.

3. *Therapeutic groups*—the nurse attempts to help the members in the social-emotional area. Emphasis is on support of positive methods and behaviors and suppression of negative methods and behaviors. Remotivation therapy is an example of a therapeutic group.

In working with groups the nurse must understand that a different type of leadership may be demanded by the objectives of the group. The different types of leadership include:

1. *Authoritarian leadership*—total power and control of the group rests with the leader whose ideas and values may be very different from the group's. This type of leadership should only be used in a crisis situation in which the objective is not changing behavior but maintaining group cohesiveness. For

example, when a member's behavior becomes so disturbed that it is upsetting to the rest of the members and interfering with group functioning and the group is unable to set limits, the leader must become the authority and ask the member to leave the group.

2. *Laissez-faire leadership*—neither power nor control of the group rests with the leader. Unless the group is very strong in its own identity and has begun to establish common goals, this type of leadership often results in complete chaos. Since anything is allowed under this type of leadership and there is free-floating of ideas, it is usually totally ineffective with psychotic patients.

3. *Democratic leadership*—the power and control of the group rests with the leader whose ideas and values are the same as the group's. The group listens and allows the leader to speak for it because the leader is symbolic of the group and is expressing its sentiments and views.

In leading a group, the nurse should try to set up a situation in which the members have something in common. The leader's objective is to develop commonalities of needs and encourage the members to express those needs that have been identified. The leader helps and encourages the group members to share their feelings. It is important that an atmosphere of full participation be maintained; therefore, group membership should be limited to ten or twelve. Creative rather than combative thinking should be fostered, and members should be encouraged to challenge those statements they cannot accept or question information that is unclear.

The leader has to recognize when periods of group silence are beneficial to provide thinking time for the members and when the silence should be interrupted. To interrupt the silence the leader can make reflective statements such as, "The group seems quiet today," or summarize group discussions that have preceded the silence. Several periods of silence usually occur in a 1-hour group meeting.

All groups usually proceed through three stages of development. In the initial or beginning phase of a group, which may last for one or three meetings, the leader must take a rather active role in setting guidelines and helping the members

111

to get to know one another. In the working phase, which may last for three or four months, the leader assumes a democratic role and gives support and encouragement to the members. In the last or termination phase, which may last for two or three meetings, the leader frequently can assume the role of an observer for by this time the members have usually found and established their own identity and need little guidance from the leader.

Study questions

1. List five things the nurse could do to make the hospital environment more like the outside community.
2. What can the nurse do to help the patient strengthen relationships with other patients?
3. How can the nurse help the patient relate to authority figures?
4. How does the nurse use the group to help individual patients?
5. List three types of groups and explain how different leadership roles could influence group functioning and achievement of goals.

Bibliography

Part I—The emotional development of man
Chapter 1—THE PARTS OF THE PERSONALITY

Brill, A.: Freud's contribution to psychiatry, New York, 1944, W. W. Norton and Co., Inc.

Erikson, E. H.: Childhood and society, New York, 1950, W. W. Norton and Co., Inc.

Freud, S.: A general introduction to psychoanalysis, Garden City, N.Y., 1943, Garden City Publishing Co.

Poland, R. G.: Human experience: a psychology of growth, St. Louis, 1974, The C. V. Mosby Co.

Sullivan, H. S.: The interpersonal theory of psychiatry, New York, 1953, W. W. Norton and Co., Inc.

Chapter 2—ESSENTIAL PERIODS IN THE FORMATION OF THE PERSONALITY

Bowers, J. E.: Caring for the elderly, Nursing **78:**42-47, January, 1978.

English, S. O., and Pearson, G. H. J.: Emotional problems of living, ed. 3, New York, 1963, W. W. Norton and Co., Inc.

Erikson, E.: Identity: youth and crisis, New York, 1968, W. W. Norton and Co., Inc.

Smith, D. W., and Bierman, E. L., editors: The biologic ages of man, Philadelphia, 1973, W. B. Saunders Co.

Snyder, J. C., and Wilson, M. F.: Elements of a psychological assessment, Am. J. Nursing **78:**235-239, 1978.

Sullivan, H. S.: The interpersonal theory of psychiatry, New York, 1953, W. W. Norton and Co., Inc.

Chapter 3—THE ROLE OF ANXIETY

Basic Systems, Inc.: Anxiety recognition and intervention, Am. J. Nurs. **65:**129-152, 1965.

Burkhardt, M.: Response to anxiety, Am. J. Nurs. **69:**2153-2154, 1969.

Selye, H.: The stress syndrome, Am. J. Nurs. **65:**97-99, 1965.

Chapter 4—THE USE OF DEFENSE MECHANISMS

Freud, A.: The ego and the mechanisms of defense, London, 1937, Hogarth Press.

Peterson, M.: Understanding defense mechanisms, Am. J. Nurs. **72:**1651-1674, 1972.

Chapter 5—COMMUNICATION

Goldin, P., and Russell, B.: Therapeutic communication, Am. J. Nurs. **69:**1928-1930, 1969.

Thompson, W. N.: Fundamentals of communication, New York, 1957, McGraw-Hill Book Co.

Walke, M. K.: When a patient needs to unburden his feelings, Am. J. Nurs. **77:**1164-1166, 1977.

Part II—The relationship between physical illness and emotional problems

Chapter 6—PATIENTS WITH EMOTIONAL PROBLEMS RESULTING FROM PHYSICAL ILLNESS

Barnard, K.: Teaching the retarded child is a family affair, Am. J. Nurs. **68:**305-311, 1968.

Cohen, S., and Rogers, T. A.: Helping depressed patients in general nursing practice, Programmed instruction, Am. J. Nurs. **77:**1007-1038, 1977.

An educational design program: understanding hostility, Am. J. Nurs. **67:**2131-2150, 1967.

Gerdes, L.: The confused or delirious patient, Am. J. Nurs. **68:**1228-1233, 1968.

Howells, J. C.: Modern perspectives in child psychiatry, Springfield, Ill., 1965, Charles C Thomas, Publisher.

Kolb, L. C.: Modern clinical psychiatry, ed. 8, Philadelphia, 1973, W. B. Saunders Co.

Oates, J.: Sexually transmitted diseases, Nurs. Times **68:**832, 1972.

Schwartz, M. S., and Shockley, E. L.: The nurse and the mental patient, New York, 1956, Russell Sage Foundation.

Sloboda, S.: Understanding patient behavior, Nursing **77:**74-77, September, 1977.

Stokes, G. A., and Fitzpatrick, P. E.: Teaching students psychotherapy, Am. J. Nurs. **77:**249-253, 1977.

Chapter 7—PATIENTS WITH PHYSICAL ILLNESS RESULTING FROM EMOTIONAL PROBLEMS

Brooks, B. R.: Aggression, Am. J. Nurs. **67:**2519-2522, 1967.

Collidge, J. C.: Asthma in mother and child as a special type of communication, Am. J. Orthopsychiatry **26:**165, 1956.

Purintun, L. R., and Nelson, L.: Ulcer patient: emotional emergency, Am. J. Nurs. **68:**1930-1933, 1968.

Ulett, G. A.: A synopsis of contemporary psychiatry, ed. 5, St. Louis, 1972, The C. V. Mosby Co.

Weiss, E., and English, S. P.: Psychosomatic medicine, Philadelphia, 1957, W. B. Saunders Co.

Wittkower, E. D., and Warnes, H., editors: Psychosomatic medicine, its clinical applications, Hagerstown, 1977, Harper & Row Publishers, Inc.

Part III—Patients with emotional disorders
Chapter 8—PATIENTS WITH PSYCHONEUROTIC DISORDERS

Cameron, N.: Personality development and psychopathology—a dynamic approach, Boston, 1963, Houghton Mifflin Co.

Fenichel, O.: The psychoanalytic theory of neurosis, New York, 1945, W. W. Norton and Co., Inc.

Mereness, D., and Taylor, C. M.: Essentials of psychiatric nursing, ed. 10, St. Louis, 1978, The C. V. Mosby Co.

Chapter 9—PATIENTS WITH PERSONALITY DISORDERS

Fredlund, D.: Juvenile delinquency and school nursing, Nurs. Outlook **18:**57-59, 1970.

Mereness, D., and Taylor, C. M.: Essentials of psychiatric nursing, ed. 10, St. Louis, 1978, The C. V. Mosby Co.

Topalis, M., and Aguilera, D. C.: Psychiatric nursing, ed. 7, St. Louis, 1978, The C. V. Mosby Co.

Chapter 10—PATIENTS WITH ADDICTIVE DISORDERS

Detzer, E., Carline, A. S., and Muller, B.: Detoxifying barbiturate addicts: hints for psychiatric staff, Am. J. Nurs. **76:**1306-1307, 1976.

Ditzler, J. M.: Rehabilitation for alcoholics, Am. J. Nurs. **76:**1772-1775, 1976.

Estes, N. J., and Heinemann, M. E.: Alcoholism: development, consequences, and interventions, St. Louis, 1977, The C. V. Mosby Co.

Huey, F. L.: In a therapeutic community, Am. J. Nurs. **71:**926-933, 1971.

Russaw, E.: Nursing in a narcotic-detoxification unit, Am. J. Nurs. **70:**1720-1723, 1970.

Ufer, L.: How to recognize and care for the alcoholic patient, Nursing **77:**37-39, October 1977.

Wiley, L., editor: Managing a hospitalized drug addict, Nursing **77:**46-51, June 1977.

Part IV—Patients with functional psychotic illnesses
Chapter 11—TOOLS UTILIZED IN PSYCHIATRIC NURSING

Anders, R. L.: When a patient becomes violent, Am. J. Nurs. **77:**1144-1148, 1977.

115

Bayer, M.: Easing mental patients' return to their community, Am. J. Nurs. **76:**406-408, 1976.

Elwell, R.: Community mental health centers, Am. J. Nurs. **70:**1014-1025, 1970.

Hitchens, E. A.: Helping psychiatric outpatients accept drug therapy, Am. J. Nurs. **77:**464-466, 1977.

Hoff, L. A.: People in crisis, understanding and helping, Menlo Park, Calif., 1978, Addison-Wesley Publishing Co.

Kesler, A. R.: Pitfalls to avoid in interviewing outpatients, Nursing **77:**70-73, September 1977.

Kyes, J., and Hofling, C. K.: Basic psychiatric concepts in nursing, ed. 3, Philadelphia, 1974, J. B. Lippincott Co.

O'Brien, M. J.: Communications and relationships in nursing, ed. 2, St. Louis, 1978, The C. V. Mosby Co.

Peplau, H.: Interpersonal relationships in nursing, New York, 1952, G. P. Putnam's Sons.

Simmons, J. A.: The nurse-client relationship in mental health nursing, ed. 2, Philadelphia, 1976, W. B. Saunders Co.

Ujheley, G.: Determinants of the nurse-patient relationship, New York, 1968, Springer Publishing Co., Inc.

Chapter 12—PATIENTS WITH SCHIZOPHRENIC
REACTIONS

Ayd, F. J.: The chemical assault on mental illness, Am. J. Nurs. **65:**70-93, 1965.

Boyajean, A.: Fighting despair, Am. J. Nurs. **78:**76-77, 1978.

Beers, C.: A mind that found itself, New York, 1908, Doubleday & Co., Inc.

Bellak, L.: Schizophrenia: a review of the syndrome, New York, 1958, Logos Press.

Bettleheim, B.: The empty fortress, New York, 1967, The Free Press.

Donner, G.: Treatment of a delusional patient, Am. J. Nurs. **69:**2642-2644, 1969.

Duran, F. A., and Errion, G. D.: Perpetuation of chronicity in mental illness, Am. J. Nurs. **70:**1707-1709, 1970.

Green, H.: I never promised you a rose garden, New York, 1964, Holt, Rinehart & Winston, Inc.

Hartman, C. C.: Psychotic mothers and their babies, Nurs. Outlook **16:**32-36, 1968.

Phinney, R. P.: The student of nursing and the schizophrenic patient, Am. J. Nurs. **70:**790-792, 1970.

Topalis, M., and Aguilera, D. C.: Psychiatric nursing, ed. 7, St. Louis, 1978, The C. V. Mosby Co.

Ulett, G. A.: A synopsis of contemporary psychiatry, St. Louis, 1972, The C. V. Mosby Co.

Chapter 13—PATIENTS WITH AFFECTIVE REACTIONS

Arieti, S., editor: Manic depressive psychosis, American Handbook of Psychiatry, vol. III, New York, 1966, Basic Books, Inc.

Ayd, F. J.: The chemical assault on mental illness—the antidepressants, Am. J. Nurs. **65:**78-84, 1965.

Kolb, L. C.: Modern clinical psychiatry, ed. 8, Philadelphia, 1973, W. B. Saunders Co.

Sumner, F. C., and Gwozda, T. A.: A nurse for suicidal patients, Am. J. Nurs. **76:**1792-1793, 1976.

White, C. L.: Nurse counseling with a depressed patient, Am. J. Nurs. **78:**437-439, 1978.

Chapter 14—REMOTIVATING THE EMOTIONALLY DISTURBED PATIENT THROUGH GROUPS

Anderson, R. E., and Carter, I. E.: Human behavior in the social environment, Chicago, 1974, Aldine Publishing Co.

Carruth, B. F.: Modifying behavior through social learning, Am. J. Nurs. **76:**1804-1806, 1976.

Fochtman, G. A.: Therapeutic factors of the informal group, Am. J. Nurs. **76:**238-239, 1976.

Marram, G. D.: The group approach in nursing practice, St. Louis, 1978, The C. V. Mosby Co.

Mills, M. B.: Learning to work in groups, New York, 1970, Teachers College Press.

Ohlsen, M. M.: Group counseling, New York, 1970, Holt, Rinehart & Winston, Inc.

Olmsted, M. S.: The small group, New York, 1959, Random House, Inc.

Glossary

affect An individual's feeling tone. This term is frequently used interchangeably with the term *emotion*.

aggression An act of force against another. This attack may be verbal, physical, or symbolic in nature.

ambivalence The coexistence in one person of opposing emotional feelings toward another person, object, or goal.

anal stage Freud's second stage of development. This stage occurs in the second year of life and is concerned with the bodily function of elimination. The child learns to tolerate frustration and begins to hold on or to let go to win the approval of significant others.

anxiety A reaction of apprehension that may range from uneasiness to complete panic, which usually follows a real or symbolic condition of threat. In many instances, the source of the danger is mainly unknown or unrecognized.

apathy A lack of interest, emotion, and feeling.

association A part of the thought process concerned with the clustering of ideas. The occurrence of one idea stimulates the occurrence of another.

associative links The mental bridges between the clustering of ideas. Frequently the bridges in the present situation act to stimulate recall of unconscious material.

autism Individualized, self-centered thought, which is unrelated to reality and which is frequently utilized to obtain the satisfactions the individual is unable to obtain from reality.

blocking A difficulty in association, where the thought or speech is interrupted in midstream and the individual cannot remember the next step. Blocking is usually the result of emotional conflict, as the person unconsciously does not want to recall the thought.

body image How individuals see their own bodies. This concept can be true and realistic or it can be distorted by the unconscious.

chemotherapy The treatment of an illness by the use of chemical substances (drugs).

coma A total loss of the conscious level. The patient cannot be awakened or aroused by external stimuli.

compulsion A repetitive act of irrational behavior that an individual is emotionally forced to carry out, although it serves no rational purpose.

confabulation An unconscious making up of stories to fill in for blanks in memory.

conflict A condition of emotional tension that may be on the conscious or unconscious level. Usually occurs as a result of opposing wishes or instincts.

confusion A clouding of the conscious level of thought.

delirium A disturbance in the conscious level of thought that results in disorientation and confusion and is usually accompanied by hallucinations, illusions, and delusions.

delusion A fixed false belief that has no basis in reality and cannot be changed by logical argument or contradictory evidence. The most common types are delusions of grandeur, delusions of persecution, and delusions or ideas of reference.

dependency A lack of self-reliance that results in the individual continually seeking the assistance and the reassurance of other people.

depression A feeling of dejection or melancholy that may reach the depth of morbid sadness. This term is usually not used when referring to the realistic grief that follows an actual loss.

disorientation A disturbance in the conscious level of thought that results in a confusion of time, place, and person.

dissociation The unconscious separation of emotionally conflicting ideas, situations, and objects from the conscious level of thought.

distortion An out-of-focus, confused view of reality that occurs as the result of emotional conflict.

emotion A subjective sensation or feeling such as love, hate, anger, sadness, or joy.

empathy An objective awareness of another person's behavior and emotions that allows the individual to feel as the other person does.

euphoria An unrealistic feeling of happiness and well-being that is unrelated to reality.

fixation The failure to move beyond an early, immature level of emotional development. This term is also used to refer to an abnormal attachment to some person or object.

flight of ideas The verbal introduction of new ideas before the previous idea has been completed.

free-floating anxiety An encompassing type of anxiety that cannot be related to a specific cause.

frustration An emotional sensation that develops when an individual is prevented from achieving a goal.

fugue state A period of total disorientation, loss of identity, and bizarre behavior. These periods may occur in patients with the diagnosis of catatonic schizophrenia.

functional psychosis A mental illness in which organic or structural changes in the brain are absent or occur after the illness has begun.

grandiose Delusions of greatness, wealth, or power.

hallucination A false sensory perception without external stimuli. Any of the five senses may be involved, but the auditory is the most frequent. Hallucinations can result from emotional factors and physical illness and can also be induced chemically by such drugs as LSD and by alcohol.

heterosexuality Sexual attraction to members of the opposite sex.

homosexuality Sexual attraction to members of the same sex.

ideas of reference Delusions that all chance remarks or glances by others relate to the individual.

illusion A misinterpretation of an actual external stimuli.

incompetency A legal term meaning an individual is unable to handle personal affairs because of mental impairment.

insane A legal term, not used medically, meaning mental derangement.

instinct The unlearned, unconditioned inner drives that are mainly concerned with the gratification of biologic needs.

interpersonal relationships The reciprocal influences that two or more persons exert on one another.

lability of mood An instability of feelings, emotions, and mood characterized by rapid shifts from one extreme to another.

latency period Freud's term for the period of emotional development between the Oedipal stage and the onset of puberty, when the interests in sex are quite dormant and decreased (usually between the ages of 5 and 12 years).

libido Freud's term for sexual energy and the drive for sexual gratification.

manic behavior Periods of frenzied excitement, hyperactivity, and unrealistic euphoria.

masturbation The self-stimulation of the genital area.

melancholia A morbid, deep depression of total affect with greatly reduced motor activity.

milieu The individual's total environment, including objects and people.

motivation The drive to behavior and the goad to action.

need A condition of unsatisfied motives. A lack or imbalance that initiates behavior aimed at the correction of this condition.

neologism Meaningless words that have meaning only to the person who coined them.

neurosis (psychoneurosis) A maladjustive type of behavior that is classified as a mental disturbance and is characterized by many fears and anxieties.

obsession A persistent drive, thought, or impulse that a person cannot erase or otherwise remove from the mind.

Oedipal stage Freud's term for that period between infancy and latency when the child develops a love attachment for the parent of the opposite sex and becomes extremely jealous of the parent of the same sex. The fear of punishment for these feelings causes their repression, and the child learns to identify with the parent of the same sex (usually 3 to 6 years).

oral stage Freud's term for the first stage of emotional development. This stage occurs in the first year of life and is concerned with the taking in through the mouth. Emotional growth is possible when the infant is fed and cared for by loving and giving parents.

organic psychosis A mental illness in which organic or structural changes in the brain are present and occur before the illness has begun.

orientation The conscious awareness of self in relation to time, place, and person.

panic The disorganized behavior that results from a state of acute fear and severe anxiety.

peer A person of the same rank or standing; an equal in any respect.

perception The awareness of sensory stimulation.

phobia A morbid fear of objects, places, or things.

psyche The mind.

psychoanalysis Freud's technique for investigating the unconscious motivations and drives of an individual. This therapy uses the past to change the present behavior.

psychosomatic The physical or organic changes produced in the body by emotional conflict. The study of the relationship between the mind (psyche) and the body (soma).

psychotherapy A form of treatment for individuals with emotional disturbances. The patient is encouraged and assisted through therapy to find more acceptable methods for responding to and reducing emotional conflict.

puberty The stage of development that marks the beginning of adolescence. Usually considered the onset of the menses in the girl and the appearance of pubic hair in the boy.

reality The environment, and all it includes, as it really exists.

recall The remembrance of a past experience.

regression A return to an earlier, more infantile level of development in an attempt to attain the gratification of unmet needs.

ritual An extremely detailed act that is repeated over and over again in its complete form.

schizoid personality The personality type characterized by nonsocial and introverted behavior.

sensorium The individual's orientation to the immediate environment.

significant figures The people with whom one has intimate relationships and who have the power to greatly influence the life-style of the individual.

soma The body.

stereotypy A purposeless, exact repetition of actions or words, almost as if they were produced by a tape recorder and film.

symbol Any sensory stimuli that produces a response originally attached to another stimuli.

sympathy A subjective feeling of sorrow for another person; it is usually noncritical and accomplishes little of lasting value.

toxic psychosis A mental illness that occurs as the result of the effects of chemicals or drugs. The chemicals can be produced by the body or taken directly into the body.

transference The unconscious attachment of emotions to individuals in the present as if they were someone in the past.

unintentional acts A consciously unintended act that serves to accomplish an unconscious wish or need. These acts are sometimes referred to as "Freudian slips."

waxy flexibility or **cera flexibilitas** The arms and legs take on a waxy consistency, and the patient offers little resistance to alterations of posture and position. This state is seen in patients with catatonic schizophrenia.

withdrawal The turning away from others and the turning into the self.

word salad A peculiar pattern of speech sometimes observed in a schizophrenic person. It is characterized by the use of words and phrases that have no logical meaning or any possible connection.

Index

A

Acceptance
    of dependency needs by nurse,
        85-86
    of hostility in care of patient with
        essential hypertension, 55
    of life roles, 17
    of patient as person by nurse, 84
Acrophobia, 62
Acting out as defense, 68
Activities for patient with affective
    reaction, 106
Acute brain disorders, 44-45
Acute schizophrenic reactions, 93-94
Addictive disorders, 70-75
Adolescence
    early, 22
    identity diffusion, 22
    pre, 22
Adulthood, 18-19, 23
    young, 23
Affect
    disturbances in
        in affective reactions, 102
        in schizophrenic reactions, 92
    lack of, phobic reactions and, 61
Affective reactions, 102-108
Aggression
    in adulthood, 19
    essential hypertension and, 55
"Agitated" state, 95
Agoraphobia, 62
Alcohol, 74
    and addictive disorders, 70-75
Alcoholic deterioration, chronic,
    48-49
Alcoholic toxicity, acute brain
    disorders and, 44-45
Alcoholics Anonymous, 72
Ambivalence, 54, 92
    love, hate, 20

Amnesia, 64
Amphetamine, 74
Amytal, sodium, 59
Anal stage, 20
Anger
    essential hypertension and, 55
    internalized
        in addictive disorders, 72
        depressive reactions and, 63-64
    nurse's response to, 41-43
    as psychic phase of illness, 41-43
Antidepressants, 108
Antihistamines, 108
Antihypertensive drugs, 108
Antirheumatic compounds, 108
Antisocial behavior, addictive
        disorders and, 70
Antisocial reactions, 67
Anxiety
    beginning, 20
    behavioral mechanisms of, 26, 28
    childhood schizophrenia and,
        89-91
    degrees of, 26, 28
    drugs or alcohol to decrease,
        70-75
    early adolescence, 20
    first experience of, 25
    "free-floating," 60
    in late teens, 18
    nurse's role in reduction of, 84
    physical illness as defense for, 41
    physical symptoms of, 26
    in psychoneuroses, 59-65
    psychosomatic illnesses and, 52-55
    role of, 25-29
    in schizophrenic reactions, 90, 92,
        94, 98
Anxiety reactions, 60
Approaches
    objective, by nurse, 84-85

123

Approaches—cont'd
  therapeutic, in nurse-patient
    relationship, 87
Arteriosclerosis, cerebral, chronic
  brain disorders and, 46-48
Association, disturbance of, 92
Asthma, 53
Attention, disturbance of, in
  schizophrenic reactions, 92
Autism, 90, 92
Autistic child, 90
Autonomic nervous system,
  psychosomatic illness and, 52
Autonomous will, 20

B

Barbiturates, 74
Beers, Clifford, 5
Behavior
  in acute brain disorders, 44-45
  antisocial, addictive disorders
    and, 70
  compulsive, ulcerative colitis and,
    54-55
  in general paresis, 48
  hyperactive, affective reactions
    and, 102-108
  psychotic, 89
Behavioral mechanisms of anxiety,
  26-28
Bethlehem Asylum, 3
Bicetre Institution for Psychiatric
  Patients, 4
Bleuler, Eugene, 5
Body image, 21
  disturbances of, 92
Bowel training, obsessive
  compulsive reactions and, 61
Brain disorders
  acute, 44-45
  chronic, 46-48
  earliest symptoms of, 44

C

Catatonic schizophrenia, 95-96
Cerebral arteriosclerosis, chronic
  brain disorders and, 46-48
Cerebral symptoms of general
  paresis, 48
Cerebral vascular changes, 46
Charcot, Jean Martin, 5
Childhood, 21
Childhood schizophrenia, 89-91
Christian period, early, care of
  mentally ill in, 2
Chronic alcoholic deterioration,
  48-49

Chronic brain disorders, 46-48
Chronic schizophrenic reactions,
  93
Circulatory disturbances, 44
Claustrophobia, 62
Climacterium, 104
Clinic nurse, 82
Cliques, 22
Cocaine, 74
Colitis, ulcerative, 54-55
Coma in acute brain disorders,
  44
Communication, 34-37
  components of, 34
  conscious and unconscious,
    34-36
  of toddler, 16
Compazine, 99
Compensation, 30
Competition, 21
Compromise, 21
Compulsions as defense in
  psychoneuroses, 61
Compulsive behavior, ulcerative
  colitis and, 54-55
Compulsive personalities, 67
Confidence as goal of infancy, 15
Conflicts
  of dependency and independency,
    obsessive compulsive
    reactions and, 61
  between internal and external
    stresses, 59
  with society, addictive disorders
    and, 70
Confusion in acute brain disorders,
  44
Congenital factors, chronic brain
  disorders and, 46
Connecticut State Society for
  Mental Hygiene, 5
Conscious communication, 34-37
Conscious level of thought, 11
Control of situation in care of
  patients with sociopathic
  personalities, 68-69
Conversion as defense in
  psychoneuroses, 62-63
Conversion reactions, 30-31, 62-63
Cooperation, 21
Cranial pressure, increased, 45
Crisis period, hospitalization during,
  79-81
Cumulative effect of
  antidepressants, 108
Curiosity and fantasy, 22
Cyclothymic personality, 66

D

Day and night care center, 82
Daydreaming, 22
Defense mechanisms, 30-33
  acting out as, 69
  compulsive behavior as, in
    ulcerative colitis, 54
  in dissociative reaction, 64
  physical illness as, 41
  in psychoneuroses, 59
  support of, during physical illness,
    43
Delirium in acute brain disorders, 44
Delusions, 44, 92, 96-97
Denial, 31
  as psychic phase of illness, 43
Dependency drugs, 74
Dependency needs, 42
  addictive disorders and, 70-75
  asthma and, 53
  conflicts between independency
    and, obsessive compulsive
    reactions in, 61
  in depressive reactions, 63-64
  nurse's role in accepting and
    meeting, 85
  peptic ulcer and, 53-54
Depressants, 74
Depression
  affective reactions and, 102-108
  as defense in psychoneurosis,
    63-64
  as psychic phase of illness, 41-43
Depressive psychosis, manic,
  102-108
Depressive reactions
  psychoneurotic, 63-64
  psychotic, 102
Despair-disgust, 24
Development
  of personality, defects in, 66
  of self-concept, 14, 15
  stages of, 14-19
Dickens, Charles, 4-5
Disorientation in acute brain
  disorders, 44
Displacement, 31
Dissocial reactions, 67
Dissociation as defense in
  psychoneuroses, 64
Dissociative reactions, 64
Dix, Dorothea Lynde, 4-5
Drugs
  and addictive disorders, 70-75
  table of, 74-75
  toxicity of, acute brain disorders
    and, 44-45

E

Eastern State Hospital, 4
Ego, 12
  integrity, 24
  poorly developed, in childhood
    schizophrenia, 90
Elavil, 108
Electroconvulsive therapy, 100-101
Emotional decline in chronic
  alcoholic deterioration, 48-49
Emotional illness, early signs of, 80
Emotional problems
  facilities for treating, 81-83
  in patients with physical illness
    resulting from, 52-55
  resulting from physical illness,
    41-51
Emotionally unstable personalities in
  personality trait disturbances,
    66-67
Emotions, disturbances in, in
  affective reactions, 85
Empathy, 20, 26
Environment
  in acute brain disorders, 44-45
  in addictive disorders, structured,
    72-74
  in anxiety reactions, 60
  in childhood schizophrenia, 90-91
  in chronic brain disorders, 46-48
  emotional problems and, 52
  for mentally deficient patients,
    49-51
  for schizophrenic patients, 94-101
  in sociopathic personality
    disturbances, 68-69
  for suicidal patients, 105
  therapeutic, 87
Equanil, 100
Erikson, Erik, 19-24
Essential hypertension, 55
Exercise for patient with chronic
  brain disorders, 47
Exhaustion, physical, in manic
  depressive psychosis, 104
Experimentation in preschool stage,
  16-17
Exploration of reality in preschool
  stage, 16-17
External and internal stresses,
  conflict between, 59

F

Families
  of childhood schizophrenic
    patients, 90
  of elderly patient, 47-48

125

Family relationships, 14-19
  disturbance of, in schizophrenic
    reactions, 91
Fantasy
  in adolescence, 22
  as defense mechanism, 31
  in preschool stage, 16
Fears
  in acute brain disorders, 44
  in adulthood, 19
  of particular objects or situations,
    61-62
  of patient, reduction of, 85
Feelings
  of guilt, depressive reaction and,
    63
  of inferiority, addictive disorders
    and, 72
  of love for parent of opposite sex,
    conversion reactions and,
    62-63
  of patient
    recognition of, 84
    understanding of, 86
  of worth in toddler stage, 15-16
  of worthlessness, depressive
    reaction and, 63
"Fight" mechanism, 55
Franklin, Benjamin, 3
Freedom and control, 21
"Free-floating" anxiety, 60
Freezone as nondependency drug,
    75
Freud, Sigmund, 4, 12, 19-24
Fugue states, 64, 95
Functional psychotic illnesses,
    77-112
  affective reactions in, 102-108
  schizophrenic reactions in, 91-101
  tools utilized in psychiatric
    nursing in, 79-88

G

Gasoline as nondependency drug, 75
General paresis, 48
Generativity, 23
Genetic factors, chronic brain
    disorders and, 46
Genital stage, 22
Glue as nondependency drug, 75
Goals
  in adulthood, long-term, 18-19
  of stages of development, 14-19
Good me—bad me concept, 20
Greece, early, care of mentally ill
    patient in, 1-2
Grieving, syndrome of, 63

Group activities for patients with
    chronic brain disorders, 47
Group therapy for addictive
    disorders, 73
Groups
  for addictive disorders, 72-73
  didactic teaching, 110
  peer, 17
  task centered, 110
  therapeutic, 110
Guidelines for psychiatric nursing,
    84-87
Guilt feelings
  absence of, in sociopathic
    personality disturbances, 67
  depressive reaction and, 63
  patients with addictive disorders
    and, 72
  in preschool stage, 16-17
  ulcerative colitis and, 54-55

H

Habits, drug, 70-75
Hairspray as nondependency drug,
    75
Hallucinations, 44, 92-97
Hallucinogens, 75
Hebephrenic schizophrenia, 97-98
Heredity, emotional problems and,
    52
Heroin, 74
Hero worship, 22
Hippocrates, 1
Home care services, 82
Hospital admission, anxiety in, 41
Hospitalization during crisis period,
    81
Hospitals
  Bethlehem Asylum, 3
  Bicetre Institution for Psychiatric
    Patients, 4
  Eastern State, 4
  facilities for treating emotional
    problems, 81-83
  Hotel Dieu, 3
  New York, 4
  Pennsylvania, 3
  York Retreat, 4
Hostility, essential hypertension
    and, 55
Hotel Dieu, 3
Hyperactive behavior
  affective reactions and,
    102-108
  in catatonic schizophrenia, 96
Hypertension, essential, 55
Hypnosis, 59

I

Id, 12
Id drives in infancy, 15
Id functioning, 20
Ideas of reference, 96
Identification as defense mechanism, 31
Identity, maintaining of, in chronic brain disorders, 47
Illness
  physical
    as defense to control anxiety, 41
    patients with emotional problems resulting from, 41-51
    resulting from emotional problems, 52-55
  psychic phases of, 41-43
Illusions, 44
Imagination, 21
Imitation in preschool stage, 17
Inadequate personality, 66
Incidence
  of schizophrenia, 91
  of suicide, 105
Independence
  in adulthood, 18-19
  as goal of toddler stage, 16
  learning, 22
  nurse's role in fostering, 85
Infancy, 14-15, 20
Infectious agents
  acute brain disorders and, 44-45
  chronic brain disorders and, 46-48
Inferiority, feelings of, addictive disorders and, 72
Injections, intramuscular, for schizophrenic patients, 99-100
Insecurity
  basic, in sociopathic personality, 68
  in early teens, 18
Insulin coma therapy, 100
Intelligence, 18-19
Interdependent relationships, formation of, 18
Internal and external stresses, conflict between, 59
Internalization of values, 17
Interpersonal behavior, aim of, 36
Interpersonal relationships, 36
  difficulty in early, 36
  in schizophrenic reactions, 91-98
Interpersonal techniques
  common errors in, 87-88
  primary goal of, 36
Intimacy, 23-24

Intramuscular injections for schizophrenic patients, 99-100
Introjection, 31-32
Involutional psychosis, 104
Isolation, 23

K

Kraepelin, Emil, 5

L

Latency period, 21
Leadership
  authoritarian, 110
  democratic, 111
  laissez-faire, 111
Learning
  how to release tension, 23
  to accept interference, 20
  to be independent, 23
  to deal with intimacy, 23
  to delay satisfaction, 20
  to use power, 20
Levels
  of behavior in acute brain disorders, 44
  of understanding in mental retardation, 51
Librium, 100
Life roles, acceptance of, 17
Limits, setting of appropriate, nurse and, 86
Listening, 36
Longer-acting antidepressants, 108
Long-term goals in adulthood, 18-19
Love
  in adulthood, 19
  lack of, phobic reactions and, 61-62
  for parent of opposite sex, conversion reactions and, 62-63
  in toddler stage, 16
  someone of same sex, 22
  someone of opposite sex, 23
LSD, 75
Lust, 22

M

Magical thoughts, 20
Major tranquilizers, 99
Manic depressive psychosis, 102-104
Marihuana, 75
Masturbation, 16
Maturity, factors in, 18-19, 21
Mechanisms
  behavioral, of anxiety, 28
  of defense, 30-33

Mechanisms—cont'd
  of defense—cont'd
    acting out as, 68
    in dissociative reaction, 64
    "fight," 55
Melancholia, 104
Mellaril, 99
Memory disturbances, 92
Menopause, 104
Mental deficiency, 49-51
Mental health, potential for growth
    toward, 86-87
Mentally ill patient, care of
    in ancient Greece, 1, 2
    in early Christian period, 2
Metabolic factors, acute brain
    disorders and, 44
Meyer, Adolph, 5
Minor tranquilizers, 100
Mistrust, 20
Mood, disturbances in, 102
Mood elevators, 108
Moral conscience control, lack of,
    67
Morality, sense of, 19
Morphine, 74
Mother substitute, nurse as, 64
Mother-child relationship, childhood
    schizophrenia and, 90
Motor or sensory functions, sudden
    impairment of, 62-63
Mouth, taking in or biting off, 20
Multiple personality, 64

N

Narcotics, 108; see also Drugs
Narcotics Anonymous, 72
Nardil, 108
National Society for Mental
    Hygiene, 5
Needs
  dependency, 42
    addictive disorders and, 70-75
    asthma and, 53
    in depressive reactions, 63-64
    nurse's role in accepting and
      meeting, 84
    peptic ulcer and, 53-54
    nurse-patient relationship in
      meeting, 85
Nervous system, autonomic, in
    peptic ulcer, 54
New York Hospital, 4
Night- and day-care center,
    82
Nondependency drugs, 75
Nonverbal communication, 34

Nurse; see also Nursing care of
    patients
  in acceptance
    and meeting dependency needs,
      85-86
    of patient as person, 84
  as authority figure, 69
  clinic, 82
  and limit setting, 86
  as mother substitute, 64
  objectivity of, 84
  and potential for growth of
    patient, 86
  in recognizing own feelings, 84
  in reduction of fears and anxieties
    of patient, 85
  response of, to anger, 41-43
  and therapeutic relationship, 84-85
    approaches in, 87
  as willing listener, 42, 84-85
Nurse Practice Act, 7
Nursing, psychiatric
  in the community, 82
  guidelines for, 84-87
  tools utilized in, 79-88
Nursing care of patients; see also
    Nurse
  with acute brain disorders, 44-45
  with addictive disorders, 72-74
  with affective disorders, 102-108
  with anxiety reactions, 60
  with asthma, 53
  with cerebral arteriosclerosis,
    46-48
  with conversion reactions, 62-63
  with depressive reactions, 63-64
  with electroconvulsive therapy,
    106-107
  with essential hypertension, 55
  with general paresis, 48
  with mental retardation, 49-51
  with obsessive compulsive
    reactions, 61
  with peptic ulcer, 53-54
  with personality pattern and
    personality trait disturbances,
    67
  with phobic reactions, 61-62
  with schizophrenic reactions,
    91-101
  with sociopathic personality,
    68-69
  with ulcerative colitis, 54-55
Nutrition
  in addictive disorders, 73
  in affective reactions, 105
  in catatonic schizophrenia, 95

Nutrition—cont'd
  chronic alcoholic deterioration
    and, 49
  chronic brain disorders and, 47

O
Objective approach by nurse, 84
Observing, 36
Obsessions as defense in
    psychoneuroses, 61
Obsessive compulsive reactions, 61
Oedipal stage, 21
One-to-one relationship for suicidal
    patient, 105
Opiates, 74
Oral stage, 20
Orientation, reality, 19
Outpatient clinic, 81-82
Overactivity
  affective reactions and, 104
  in catatonic schizophrenia, 96

P
Pactal, 108
Paranoid personality, 66
Paranoid schizophrenia, 96-97
Paresis, general, 48
Parnate, 108
Passive aggressive personalities,
    66-67
Patients
  with addictive disorders, 70-75
  with affective reactions, 102-108
  with emotional problems resulting
    from physical illness, 41-51
  with functional psychotic
    illnesses, 77-112
    tools utilized in psychiatric
      nursing for, 79-88
  with personality disorders, 66-69
  as persons, nurse's acceptance of,
    84
  with physical illness resulting
    from emotional problems,
    52-55
  with psychoneurotic disorders,
    59-65
  recognition of feelings of, 84
  reduction of fears and anxieties
    of, 85
  return to community, 81
  with schizophrenic reactions,
    91-101
    nursing care of, 94-101
  therapeutic approaches in nurse's
    relationship to, 84-85
  understanding feelings of, 84

Pattern disturbances in personality,
    66
Peer group, 17, 21
Pennsylvania Hospital, 3
Peptic ulcer, 53-54
Personality
  defects in development of, 66
  degeneration of, in general
    paresis, 48
  disintegrated, 91
  multiple, 64
  parts of, 11-13
  pathologic trends in structure of,
    66
  periods in formation of, 14-19
  prepsychotic, in involutional
    psychosis, 104
  self-centered, 68
Personality disorders, 66-69
Personality disturbances
  addictive, 70
  pattern, 66-67
  trait, 66-67
Phases of illness, psychic, 41-43
Phobias as defense in
    psychoneuroses, 61-62
Phobic reactions, 61-62
Physical exhaustion in manic
    depressive psychosis, 104
Physical illness
  as defense to control anxiety, 41
  from emotional problems, 52-55
  patients with emotional problems
    resulting from, 41-51
Physical symptoms of anxiety, 26
Pinel, Phillipe, 4
Plato, 2-3
Play age, 21
Postpartum psychosis, 98
Prepsychotic personality in
    involutional psychosis, 104
Preschool as stage of development,
    16-17, 21
Pressure, increased cranial, 45
Preteen stage of development, 17-18
Projection, 32
Protection of schizophrenic patient,
    96
Psychiatric nursing; see also Nurse;
    Nursing care of patients
  guidelines for, 84-87
  tools utilized in, 79-88
Psychic phases of illness, 41-43
Psychoneurotic disorders, 59-65
Psychosis
  affective reactions and, 102-108
  involutional, 104

129

Psychosis—cont'd
  manic depressive, 102-104
  postpartum, 98
  schizophrenic reaction as, 91-101
  tools utilized in psychiatric
    nursing in, 79-88
Psychosomatic illnesses, 52-55
Psychotherapy, 59
  for addictive disorders, 73
Psychotic behavior, 89
Psychotic depressive reactions, 102
Psychotic illnesses; see Psychosis

R
Rationalization, 32
Reaction-formation, 32
Reactions
  affective, 102-108
  conversion, 30-31
  dissocial or antisocial, 67
  psychoneurotic, 59-65
  psychotic depressive, 102
  schizophrenic, 91-101
Reality
  exploration of, in preschool stage,
    16-17
  orientation to, 18
Regression, 32
Rejection
  of patient, 84
  in toddler stage, 15-16
Relationships
  with asthmatic patient, 53
  family, 14-19
    disturbance of, in schizophrenic
      reactions, 91
  interdependent, formation of, 18
  interpersonal, 36
    early, difficulty in, 36
    in schizophrenic reactions,
      91-101
  therapeutic approaches in
    nurse-patient, 87
  mother-child, childhood
    schizophrenia and, 90-91
  one-to-one, for suicidal patient,
    105
  with opposite sex, establishment
    of, 18
  between physical illness and
    emotional problems, 41-51,
    59-65
Remotivation, social, 109
Repetitive thoughts and actions, 61
Repression, 32-33
  in dissociative reaction, 64
Respect for patient as person, 84

Retardation, mental, 49-51
Rituals, 61
Role
  of anxiety, 25-29
  heterosexual, 22
  homosexual, 22
  identity, 21
  of life, acceptance of, 17
  social, 21
Rush, Dr. Benjamin, 3

S
Safety of environment for suicidal
    patient, 105
Saint Augustine, 2
Schizoid personality, 66
Schizophrenia, 91-101
  childhood, 89-91
School age, early, in stages of
    development, 17, 21
Schools for mentally deficient
    persons, 50-51
Secondary symptoms in
    schizophrenic reactions, 92
Security
  lack of, phobic reactions and,
    61-62
  in peer group as goal of early
    school period, 17
Sedatives, 74
Self-centered personality, 68
Self-concept, development of, 14, 15
Self control, 20
Senescence, 24
Senility, 46-47
Sensory or motor functions, sudden
    impairment of, 62-63
Sex role, 21-22
Shame and doubt, 20
Short-acting antidepressants, 108
Side effects
  of antidepressants, 108
  of tranquilizers, 99
Significant others, 21
Simple schizophrenia, 94-95
Sleepwalking, 64
Social achievement, 21
Social controls, chronic alcoholic
    deterioration and, 49
Society, addictive disorders and
    conflict with, 70
Society of Friends, 3
Sociopathic personality
    disturbances, 67-69
Sodium amytal, 59

Solvents as nondependency drugs, 75
Sparine, 99
Speech, changes in, 92
Stages of development, 14-19
Stelazine, 99
Steroids, 108
Stimulants, 74
Stresses
  conflict between internal and external, 59
  inability to handle, addictive disorders and, 70
  in schizophrenic reactions, 91-101
Structure of personality, pathologic trends in, 66
Stupor, 44-45, 95
Subconscious level of thought, 11
Sublimation, 33
Suicide, prevention of, 105
Sullivan, Harry S., 19-24
Superego, 13
  development, 21
  lack of, 67
  in preschool stage, 17
Support during crisis, 80
Suppression, 33
Survival, 20
Symbiosis, 20
Symptoms
  of addictive disorders, 74
  of affective reactions, 102-104
  of anxiety, physical, 26
  of anxiety reactions, 60
  of brain disorders, earliest, 44
  of childhood schizophrenia, 89-91
  of chronic alcoholic deterioration, 49
  of chronic brain disorders, 46-48
  of conversion reactions, 62-63
  of crisis, 80
  of depression, 42-43
  of depressive and dissociative reactions, 63-64
  of early emotional illness, 79
  of general paresis, 48
  of personality disorders, 67-69
  of phobic reactions, 61-62
  of psychoneuroses, 59
  of schizophrenic reactions, 91-98
Syndrome of grieving, 63-64
Syphilis, 48

T

Tasks of growth periods, 19-24
Teens in stages of development, 18

Temper tantrums, 20
Therapeutic environment, 87
Therapeutic relationships, 84-85
  approaches in, 87
Thorazine, 99
Thought levels
  conscious, 11
  subconscious, 11
  unconscious, 11-12
Toddler stage of development, 15-16, 20
Tofranil, 108
Toxic agents, chronic brain disorders and, 46
Trait disturbances in personality, 66-67
Tranquilizers, 59
  in affective disorders, 108
  in schizophrenic reactions, 99
Transference, 33
  of feelings of anxiety and hostility to symbolic object or situation, 61-62
Trauma, brain disorders and
  acute, 44
  chronic, 46
Treponema pallidum, 48
Trust, 20
Tuke, William, 4
Tumors, chronic brain disorders and, 46

U

Ulcerative colitis, 54-55
Ulcers, peptic, 53-54
Unconscious communication, 34-35
Unconscious level of thought, 11-12
Understanding
  level of, in mental retardation, 50-51
  of patient's feelings, nurse's role in, 84

V

Validation
  consensual, 22
  group, 22
Valium, 100
Values, internalization of, 17
Verbal communication, 34
Vesprin, 99
Vitamin deficiency in chronic alcoholic deterioration, 49
Voluntary admission, 81

W
Waxy flexibility, 95
Withdrawal
  in childhood schizophrenia, 90-100
  in schizophrenic reactions, 91
Worthlessness, feelings of,
    depressive reactions and,
    63-64
Writing, changes in, 92

Y
York Retreat, 4

Z
Zoophobia, 62